Pig Production

Pig Production

R. M. Acharya
B.V.Sc. & A.H. (Pb), M.S. (Ohio), Ph.D. (Iowa)
Former Deputy Director General (Animal Science) ICAR
784, Sector-9, Faridabad (Haryana)

and

Puneet Kumar, Ph.D.
Principal Scientist (Animal Physiology)
Indian Veterinary Research Institute, Izatnagar (UP)

SSPH

SATISH SERIAL PUBLISHING HOUSE
403, Express Tower, Commercial Complex
Azadpur, Delhi-110033 (India)
Phone : 011-27672852, Fax : 91-11-27672046
e-mail : info@satishserial.com, hkjain1975@yahoo.com
Website : www.satishserial.com

Published by :

SATISH SERIAL PUBLISHING HOUSE
403, Express Tower, Commercial Complex, Azadpur, Delhi-110033 (INDIA)
Phone : 011-27672852 Fax : 91-11-27672046
E-mail : info@satishserial.com, hkjain1975@yahoo.com

Reprint, 2020

ISBN 978-93-86200-14-3

Composed, Designed & Printed in India

Preface

Sustainable development is that which meets the needs of the present without compromising the ability of the future generations to meet their own needs. Since the onset of industrial era, man has been exploiting the natural resources viz. land, water, plants, animals and aquatic resources without consideration of the need of their conservation and sustainable management and the adverse effects their excessive utilization is having on soil and environmental degradation and increasing impact on the health and production of all living organisms. There is therefore a need to be more pragmatic in utilizing the natural and manmade resources and ensure their continuous availability on a sustainable basis. The impact on environment, as mentioned earlier, is a very serious issue and is currently attracting attention of the world community but little concrete steps have been taken for the diversion from the use of fossil fuels to renewable energy resources. The conventional resources are continued to be used extensively. Incentives are being provided for the conservation of natural resources but the impact especially in the industrially advanced developed countries where the use of fossil fuels is increasing is minimum. Further intensive crop production, monoculture, and use of excessive production inputs especially chemicals viz. fertilizers, pesticides and weedicides and energy resources in the form of petroleum products are leading to serious environmental consequences. For the last fifty years there has been a slogan to have integrated plant nutrient management (INM) and integrated plant pest management (IPM) and have integrated farming systems having a proper balance of crops, livestock, fish and agro-forestry. But these have made a small impact. The integrated farming system is not only required for the soil and environmental conservation but also to meet the timber and fuel needs of human society. The integrated area development approach management earlier taken up under intensive crop and livestock production programmes was to ensure that the natural resources viz soil, water and plant and animal are conserved and are sustainably utilized and there is no further deterioration in the environment and erosion of plant, animal, aquatic and microbial genetic resources. The impact, however; has been marginal. The current five year plan has emphasized more on increasing production while ensuring sustainability of natural resources.

Of the livestock, ruminants both large ruminants (cattle and buffalo) and small ruminants (sheep and goat) are the dominant species in numbers and spread and their contribution to food and nutrition and employment and incomes, particularly in rural and peri-urban areas in developing Asian countries like India. The utilization of livestock products and services is rapidly increasing because of a fast increase in human population and a large proportion of it being now moving to urban areas because of better facilities of education, employment and incomes. Further nuclearization of families is leading to an increasing demand for foods of higher quality, both nutritionally and in taste and also having a higher satiety factor. In western countries there is a gradual decline in consumption of red meat (beef and mutton) and there is a greater preference for chicken, pork and rabbit meat. This trend may also arise in India and pig may attain a greater importance in livestock production, particularly for meat in future.

Pig is a very efficient in conversion of relatively low quality feed ingredients into high quality protein food which is acceptable to most meat consumers. Although in India Muslims, the second dominant religious community and also majority of other communities which are otherwise vegetarian, have little consumption of pork. Pork is still a dominant meat among the economically and socially deprived communities who raise a few piglets under free range scavenging conditions and sell them for income or slaughter them on festive occasions for their own self consumption of meat. In spite of some efforts by the Central and State Governments in introducing exotic breeds of pigs to be raised as purebreds on the institutional farms for production of purebred or crossbred boars for grading up of indigenous pigs, the total production of pig meat has not shown any serious increase.

Livestock sector in India, as mentioned earlier, is playing an increasingly important role in providing food and nutrition, energy, industrial raw materials and sustainable self-employment and incomes, especially for economically and socially deprived rural people, like small and marginal farmers and landless laborers. Foods of livestock origin are nutritionally better balanced and contain high quality protein with essential amino acids and also possess micro-nutrients, viz. vitamins and minerals. Further, animal foods are more balanced, have higher taste and satiety factor.

Inspite of a significant growth of livestock sector in India, specially related to milk production, the meat and fiber production sectors have not grown as fast as milk sector except the buffalo meat which has both a large internal and export market and which is growing at a rapid rate. Dairy animals and chicken, the latter for meat and eggs have been given a relatively larger emphasis in research and development efforts especially because of the involvement of private sector in poultry production which has collaboration of the important international poultry breeding concerns. This involves importation of high producing genetic stocks (strains/inbred lines) and their utilization in producing hybrid layer and broiler chicks. Now, excellent performing day old chicks of broiler and layer strains and strain crosses are being marketed throughout the urban and peri-urban areas. The poultry sector especially the meat component is growing faster than any other livestock sector. Poultry, both layer and broilers, has higher reproductive efficiency and feed conversion ratio. Poultry production can be carried out in urban and peri-urban areas as the disposal of farm waste does not have serious environmental consequences and can be easily used as a feed component for ruminant livestock after proper processing and in an appropriate proportion with other concentrates and roughage inputs. Next to the chicken comes other avian species like quail and duck which have some advantages over the chicken as well as disadvantages. Next in prolificacy, growth and feed conversion efficiency comes rabbits followed by pigs.

Pig, as mentioned earlier, has been essentially considered as a scavenging animal in India and is currently raised with little production and health inputs. It is a common practice to maintain one or two breeding sows with or without a boar and in the case of latter utilize the boar from the neighboring herd and when they farrow, the piglets are large enough to fend for themselves, the owner leaves a few of them at different places to utilize household wastes and other natural feed resources available in the region. The owner only visits to ensure that the piglets are healthy and have not been predated or stolen. After they reach market weight or there is a market demand, he disposes them off. Semi-intensive and intensive rearing is not common; however, the Central and State Governments maintain pig farms with exotic breeds to produce boars for distribution to pig farmers for grading their indigenous pigs. This results in some improvement in body size and reproductive efficiency and survival. In such cases, the pigs are generally raised under scavenging conditions during the day and are housed during the night and are provided with some household waste food materials. Intensive pig production is also being done utilizing commercial feed, health care and proper housing and management. This is however generally confined to the Government farms or a few large institutional herds raised for research and education. Most of the people who raise pigs belong to the scheduled castes, scheduled tribes and other economically and socially deprived classes. Since pigs under scavenging conditions consume all kind of human waste, they are likely to transmit zoonotic diseases and thus the pig meat is not normally consumed by those people who can afford lamb/mutton/chevon/ chicken. Beef and kine (buffalo meat) are also restricted in consumption both socially and regionally.

Pig, as stated earlier, is otherwise an efficient meat producer and can have two to three liters per year, each with ten to twelve piglets and with a good average daily gain, efficiency of feed conversion and carcass yield and quality. Sows are good mothers with a large number of teats and can rear a large litter under proper feeding and management conditions. Utilizing genetically superior breeds, pork production can be highly profitable. Pigs further do not require very costly and environmentally controlled housing facilities like commercial layer/ broiler chicken and can utilize large quantities of agricultural wastes, agro-industrial byproducts and slaughter-house byproducts. Indigenous pigs generally tend to dig to burrow themselves to keep cool and it is essential that the housing facility should not allow them to burrow themselves. Similarly the houses must be provided with a guard wire/ railing so that the piglet can avoid being crushed by their mother.

Pig research and development in India is still in a nascent stage relative to other species of livestock. The ICAR had instituted an AICRP on Pigs with a coordinating unit at the Indian Veterinary Research Institute (IVRI), Izatnagar, U.P. The project envisaged raising pigs under intensive feeding and management and involved a number of exotic breeds and aimed at their improvement through selection and hybridization. The aim was to improve the litter size, litter survival, live weight gains, efficiency of feed conversion and carcass yield and quality. The project was subsequently changed to study indigenous non-descript free range scavenging pigs, both under extensive and intensive management conditions and take up their genetic improvement through selection and hybridization utilizing both indigenous and exotic breeds and additive and non-additive genetic variances in economic characters. The project now aims at improving both the exotic and indigenous breeds of pigs and also undertakes their crossing. The ICAR has more recently established a National Research Center (NRC) on Pigs at Rani, near Guwahati, Assam, which is undertaking fundamental and applied research on different aspects of swine production, developing sustainable management and conservation technologies for indigenous breeds / types and coordinating the multi-locational and multi-disciplinary project on pig production.

In the Western countries, pig is now becoming an increasingly important source of meat, because of high productivity under intensive production management in urban and peri-urban areas, requiring relatively lesser space and causing a relatively less environmental, pollution problems than ruminant livestock species which depend on large quantities of roughages. There are ethnic groups which like pig meat specially meat of black pigs and there is a growing demand for processed meat products like bacon and sausages in fast food joints. There is likelihood that with an increased urbanization, education, employment, incomes and nuclearization of families, the demand for livestock products including pig both pork and bacon and other processed products would increase.

Pig is a very clean animal and does not like to eat any soiled feed but the way pigs are maintained, under essentially scavenging conditions, they have been given a bad name of a dirty animal and spreading human diseases through consumption of its meat or through contact with the people who raise pigs essentially under scavenging conditions.

There is a need to educate, both the producers and the consumers regarding hygienic pig meat production and ensuring its quality. There is a need for the meat industry being involved in processing realizing the economic, social and nutritional importance of pig meat and undertake intensive research, education and extension activity to develop more modern production, protection, and processing technologies for intensive pig production in the country. The current research on description, evaluation, and sustainable management and conservation of different breeds and types of pigs available in the country as well as pooling all the knowledge available nationally and internationally on the pig breeds, and undertaking their genetic improvement and sustainable utilization for economic pig production along with their feeding, management and health interventions, determining appropriate age and weight at slaughter to maximize economic returns and producing quality meat for consumption as unprocessed or processed meat are areas requiring immediate R&D support.

With growing concern about soil and environmental conservation, the role of pig in degradation of soil and environment and steps that are needed to be taken to avoid such adverse contribution through appropriate management of pigs and disposal of pig farm wastes. The latter is more important in more intensive rearing of pigs and the disposal of manure should be given due importance. The socio-economic aspects of different crop-livestock-fish integrated farming systems and their impact on environment are more important issues being gradually realized both by the livestock keepers and R&D agencies and must continue to be given increasing attention and opportunities for their amelioration for ensuring sustainability of pig production in the country.

The book is based on an extensive review of literature available in the country on various aspects of pig production, health and products technology and the current limitations and the opportunities for increasing pig production both as an economic activity and as a source of protective food. The current R&D efforts, their strength and weaknesses and what more needs to be done and how the R&D should be organized so that pig production can be economically feasible and socially acceptable and can generate production technologies which would be acceptable to the pig keepers in India at present and in the foreseeable future areas are required urgent concentration by R&D. The book is expected to be used in undergraduate and postgraduate teaching and identifying research priorities and laying down a roadmap for sustainable pig production under various agro-ecological and socio-economic conditions, currently prevailing in the country and that are likely to arise in the near future.

The senior author as a Former Deputy Director General (Animal Science), Indian Council of Agricultural Research has a long experience in Education, Research and Development both at National and International level, has reviewed the present R&D activities and indicated the effectiveness of the state of knowledge of various problems related to production, health and processing technologies of pigs and has also indicated the future strategies for pig research and development in the country. On the basis of an extensive review, visits and discussions with scientists of the National Research Center on Pigs and the scientists at IVRI, the author has prepared the manuscript with the assistance of co-author Dr Puneet Kumar, Principal Scientist at the Indian Veterinary Research Institute, Izatnagar.

The book is dedicated to the socio-economically deprived people who maintain pigs for their very existence and any positive intervention which will improve pig production and thus their economic conditions will go a long way in poverty alleviation which is the most important objective of the present Government and also to ensure sufficient quantity of quality food and nutrition without causing problems of ecological degradation and ensuring sustainable economic development. The book will also help both the undergraduate and post graduate students in Veterinary and Animal Science and will provide the knowledge to the development personal engaged in promoting pig production in the country as well as private entrepreneurs who are engaged in promoting pig production or are themselves raising pigs for commercial purposes. The help rendered during the visits to National Research Centre on Pigs and ICAR-IVRI for discussions and collection of latest information has helped in bringing a more up-to-date state of knowledge and is gratefully acknowledged.

Dr. R.M.Acharya
Dr. Puneet Kumar

List of Tables

Contents

CHAPTER-1

Current Pig Production Scenario in the Country

Pig (Sukur in Sanskrit and Sur in common language) is considered a relatively dirty animal, but if bred and maintained in more intensive manner, through providing proper housing, feed and health cover can produce high quality meat very efficiently.

The current pig production system in large part of the country is essentially based on zero input (ZIP) or extremely low input (LIP). In the latter, only household food wastes and some hotel/restaurant food waste, fruit and vegetable market waste are provided. In medium input production system especially involving graded indigenous pigs with exotic breeds are provided with agro-industrial processing byproducts and food wastes from household, vegetable and fruit markets.

Indigenous pigs are relatively small in size with long snout which helps them to dig the ground to pick up food of vegetable and animal origin such as insects. The current pig genetic resources have not been subjected to any critical study and further subjected to improvement through selection or introduction of superior exotic inheritance except to a limited extent through the various pig research and development programs of the Central and State Animal Husbandry Departments and ICAR research institutes and SAUs/ SVUs. Relatively low performance and restricted consumption of pig meat have been major constraints in undertaking research and development activities for improving pig production in India. The poor performance in terms of reproduction rate, young survival, growth rate, low carcass yield and meat quality are factors which have been impeding pig development in the country. The meat of indigenous pigs is otherwise lean, with low fat content, and is liked by people who raise pigs and especially in north-eastern region.

Intensive pig production through raising exotic breeds mostly of European and American in origin, has been taken up in a few places such as in Ghaziabad in Uttar Pradesh (UP) where the UP Government had established a large exotic pig breeding farm and also established slaughter and meat processing facility and high quality pork and bacon products are produced. Some private entrepreneurs have also gone in for intensive pig production with exotic breeds for producing quality pork and bacon.

Pig production can have an important role in livelihood (employment and incomes) security and food and nutrition of people, if the stresses and shocks generally observed are removed and resources in terms of training to the people, servicing pig producers and the pig producers themselves and other inputs like cheap feed and heath cover are provided. However while intensifying production, the environmental conservation and livelihood and nutritional security of poor people who are generally associated with pig production in India, should be kept in view. Of the regions in the country, the North-East Hill region both in terms of numbers, genetic variants, production types and intensity of production and consumption of pork is the most important. In addition to providing high quality food with balanced nutrients and taste, indigenous pigs provide high quality manure and bristles. Pig dung can be used as excellent manure and before it is used as a plant nutrient, it could also be used for growing phyto-and zoo-planktons and thus help in increasing fish production. In fact crop, livestock, and fish production can be integrated to benefit from the waste of each other and to have more sustainable economic and environmentally sound production system. Pig, among different domestic animal (DA) species, can be considered as very efficient meat producer because of (i) high prolificacy (number of litters per year and number of piglet per litter), (ii) tendency to consume a wide variety of feeds of animal and plant origin, (iii) high feed conversion efficiency, (iv) relatively early age at sexual maturity, (v) short generation interval, and (vi) relatively small space required for housing.

Pig is a multipurpose animal as in addition to basic production of meat, it provides cooking fat, bristles and organic manure. It can be maintained under highly variable management systems ranging from zero input scavenging system, to the provision of night shelter and some supplementary household waste, and further to an extremely intensive and most efficient production system under confinement and intensive feeding. There is, however; some serious zoonotic problems contributed by pig primarily resulting from the way the pigs are reared in the country.

Pigs are most intelligent of the domestic animals and are being used as a model for studying human intelligence and diseases. Pigs are being developed as donors for organs for replacement in human beings. Pigs are small in size and further miniature pigs are now being evolved probably for use as model for human intelligence and health studies and provision of organs for replacement in human beings. Pigs unlike poultry can be fed more fibrous feed. Pork is a good source of animal protein for human consumption with a more balanced essential amino-acids (Arginine 6.4%, Leucine 7.5 %, Lysine 7.8%, Threonine 5.1%, Valine 5%). Pork is a rich source of poly-unsaturated fatty acids (PUFA) compared to beef, lamb, chevon or even milk, contains fatty acid - Palmitic acid 28%, Oleic acid 40%, Stearic acid 13%, Linolenic acid 10%, Cholesterol 61% which is lower than butter and other animals' meats. Pork contains higher quantity of water soluble vitamins. Pork is palatable, delicious, tender, juicy with favorable color and aroma and is liked as such or in various products especially bacon and sausages.

There is no organized marketing system of live pigs, pork and pig by-products. Local traders buy pigs for sale from the pig producers mostly based on their numbers rather than on size and live weight and sell those to the butchers for slaughter at much higher rate. There is hardly any regulated slaughter facilities of pigs, proper ante and post-mortem examination and classification of meat according to various cuts and quality. There are no cold storage facilities for pig meat.

There is a need to develop proper strategies for improvement of pig production in India both for the resource poor communities and urban intensive management for providing high quality pork and bacon to the urban population. As mentioned earlier, there is an increasing consumption of pig meat in western countries and it is also becoming a relatively dominant meat in developing countries especially in South-East Asia and China because of relatively higher ill effects of consuming red meat. The intensification of pig production, both in the rural and peri-urban areas under more intensive / semi-intensive production systems, as well as highly intensive commercialized production system need to be developed. This will involve on priority in the following components:

1.1 Feeding strategies

Identification of feed resources especially non-conventional in nature, readily available at a relatively low cost and which are not currently used by other DA species especially dairy animals and poultry and their proper compounding so that their intake, digestibility and utilization can be improved. Agro-industrial processing by-products, leaf meals, roots and tubers like Cassava, Colocasia and Azolla etc. which are not extensively used presently for human consumption or even for production of other DAs can be utilized for pig feeding.

1.2 Housing and strategies for management

There is a little protection provided to the pigs especially indigenous or even their grades with exotic breeds under more extensive production system in rural and peri-urban areas. The non-provision of proper management especially to the young piglets results in high morbidity and mortality. Cheap shelters using locally available construction materials can be built to keep the animals comfortable and protect them from extremes of weather and predation. This will improve the economics of pig production. It will also help in better management of manure.

1.3 Breeding strategies

Little is known about the indigenous breeds with respect to their positive attributes and limitations in production. Except for some efforts in undertaking surveys for description and evaluation of indigenous types of pigs by the NBAGR, NRC Pig and earlier by AICRP Pig centers, which also had serious limitation, as no long-term studies on their performance under different production systems and identifying constraints and developing suitable ameliorating measures, has been taken up. Genetic improvement for maximizing efficiency of meat production through selection within indigenous breeds, grading relatively low producing breeds of pigs with superior indigenous breeds or superior exotic breeds needs to be intensified. Some information in this regard is available from AICRP on Pigs which had operated since 1971 and had a number of centers spread in most of the important agro-ecological regions. The knowledge available on the genetic architecture both at physical, gross performance, molecular level and developing proper breeding strategies is still lacking.

1.4 Institutional support

As mentioned earlier there has been a limited R&D effort by the Central and State Governments and the ICAR and SAUs / SVUs and the State Animal Husbandry Departments. This, however; has led to some understanding of the prospects of the pig production in the country, limitations impeding the efficiency of the pig production and intervention that can be made to improve it. The application of such innervations under the current pig production system have however serious limitations.

Integrating pig production with crops; crops and fish; crops and poultry; poultry-fish and crops; rabbits, poultry, fish and crops and with other DAs, are some of the efforts to intensify pig production and ensuring proper recycling of the wastes of one component of the system as a feed stock for the production of other component which can help in improving the economics of the production as well as environmental sustainability through proper recycling of farm wastes.

Pig production can help in poverty alleviation, women empowerment, economic development of under privileged communities and providing excellent food and some by-products such as bristles and manure. Pig keepers can constitute themselves into producer group for maintaining a piglet producing unit on scientific lines using genetically superior indigenous / exotic / their crosses with proper technical and management input support and provide quality piglets to the members to be raised for collective sale at an appropriate weight / age and at an appropriate marketing opportunity. Such piglets can be collected and marketed in larger numbers at better remunerative prices. If the organization is large and the number of piglets is sufficient to support establishment of a slaughter facility and meat processing unit, it can further help in increasing shelf life and adding value to the meat and thus improving economics of pig production. Training of pig producers in scientific pig production is one serious limitation in current pig production in the country. The SAUs / SVUs and State Animal Husbandry Departments can help in training pig producers in scientific pig production as well as ensuring provision of production and health inputs and services for improving pig production. This may be in the form of better stock, compounded feed, health cover and marketing.

Pig production helps in nutrient recycling especially crop by-products and other agricultural and industrial by-products and wastes, in nutrient concentration through providing high quality cost efficient meat from those low quality nutrient resources. It can help in diversification of livestock production when it is included as a component of integrated farming system with crops, livestock and fish. It can help in improving soil structure and fertility through its high quality manure.

Pig production is economically viable and can be an important source of livelihood (employment and incomes) and food and nutritional security. The major issue is to integrate pig production in the current rural livelihood and income generation in agricultural and DA production systems and removal of the taboo on the consumption of the pig meat.

Pigs in India, as mentioned earlier, are generally raised under extensive management, mostly under scavenging condition with little supplementary feed, provision of housing / shelter / protection from inclement weather and provision of any health cover. Most of the pig keepers in rural and peri-urban areas maintain one or two sows and get them bred from a common boar which is also not changed often resulting in extensive inbreeding and its adverse effects on reproduction and survival. The age at first litter is generally high and litter performance in terms of size, survival and growth is relatively low. This is primarily due to hardly any selection / genetic improvement through introduction of superior indigenous / exotic inheritance except in highly limited locations where the Animal Husbandry Departments have taken pig production programs. These essentially involve distribution of exotic / graded male piglets to be raised as boars and used for breeding indigenous / graded sows for improving reproduction, survival, live weight gains, carcass yield and quality of their progeny. Pig production being essentially in the hands of economically, socially and culturally deprived people who have relatively low education and access to institutional finance and extension services and cannot afford superior germplasm and following improved production practices and thus cannot fully benefit from pig production. Under the various poverty alleviation and rural development programs, institutional finance at low interest rates is being provided but since most pig keepers are poor of the poorest, have little source of information on these financial resources and on the government pig development programs and further do not have knowledge about improved production practices, and thus do not benefit either from the improved production system or institutional financial support. Non-availability of institutional finance and marketing facilities further cause reluctance in adopting any improved production technology. These constraints need to be studied with respect to their prioritization and R&D and extension efforts should be intensified to remove these production constraints. These efforts should be further supported through proper education and training and provision of appropriate inputs and services. Processing and marketing are further limiting factors in improving pig production under the present scenario and must be given appropriate attention.

1.5 Pig population statistics

The population of pig has been continuously rising from 1961 to 1997 when it showed a relatively slow growth, the challenges to reverse the population growth as reflected either by the poor economics of pig production or serious production constraints especially pig diseases, there has been a large destruction of pigs because of transmission of some newly emerging viral diseases in pigs to human, however; considering the importance of pigs for tribal and certain ethnic groups and more particularly in North-Eastern Hill region, there is a need for further intensification of R&D.

As per the current (19th) Livestock Quinquennial Census-2012, the total pig population in the country has decreased by 7.54% over the previous census (2007) and the total pigs (indigenous and exotic) in the country are 10.29 million in 2012 (Fig.1) which constitutes only 1.05 % of the world pig population of 977.27m The majority of pig population in the world is in China (48.71%), followed by USA (6.63%), Brazil (4.00%), Germany (2.83%) and Vietnam (2.69%). Pigs constitute only 2.01% of the total DA population (Fig.2.) and contribute only 0.95% of the global share in pig meat production. Even in Asia, while in other DAs especially in cattle and buffaloes, it does not rank even in the first five. In Asia, India has only 1% and China 80% of the pig population. It has however been increasing, though gradually since 1947 when the country became independent of the British rule and the large part both on the West and East of the country went to constitute an independent country Pakistan. The eastern part has now become an independent country, Bangladesh. The pig population had a positive trend except during 1961-66 and 2004-2012. The maximum growth was during 1992-2003. During the last quinquennial, there was a decline in 4.47%.

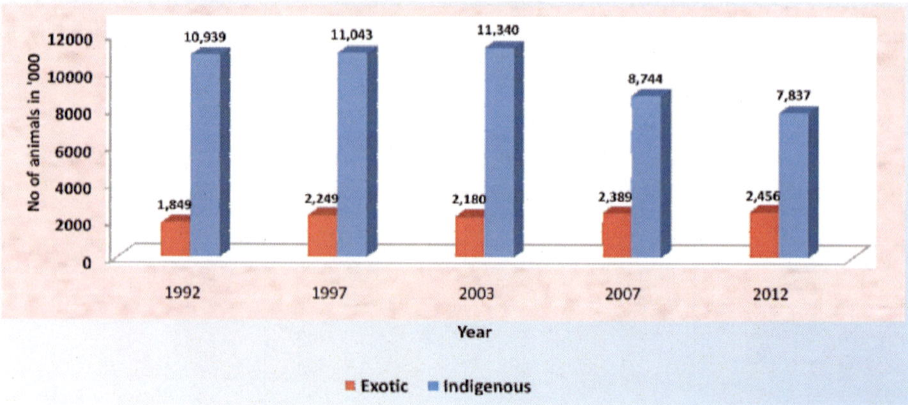

Fig. 1. Total number of pigs (indigenous and exotic) in India during 1992-2012
(*Source:* 19th Livestock Census-2012, Government of India)

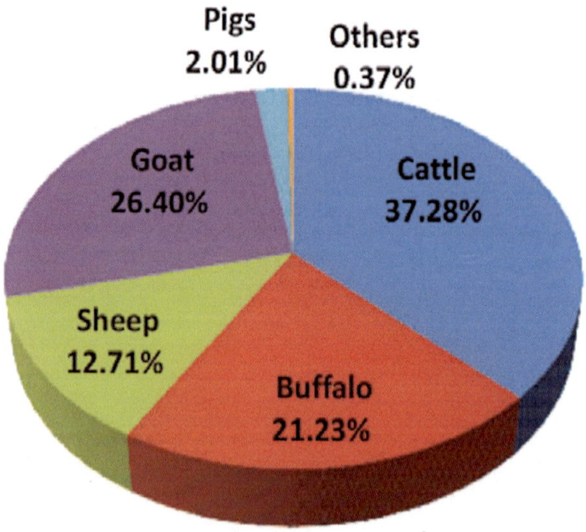

Fig. 2. Distribution of livestock in India
(*Source:* 19th Livestock Census-2012, Government of India)

The state wise pig population in India is given in Fig.3. The state of Assam has the maximum share (15.89%), whereas; the state of Rajasthan has minimum share (2.31%) of the total population of pigs in India.

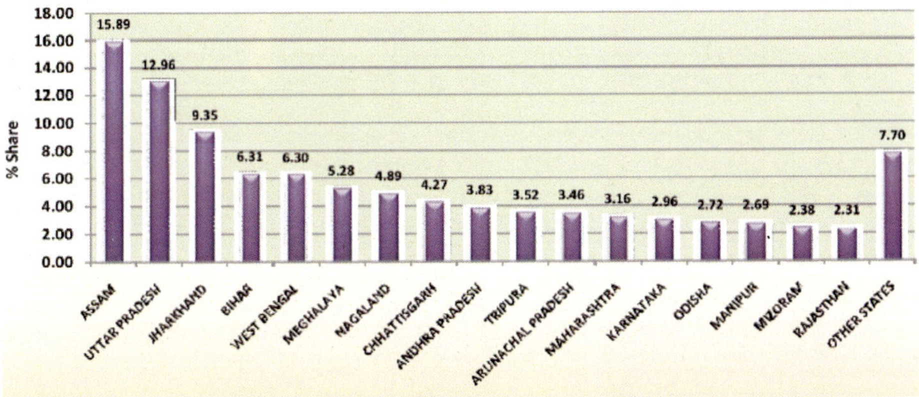

Fig. 3. State wise pig population in India
(*Source:* 19th Livestock Census-2012, Government of India)

Percent change in the population of pigs from 2007 to 2012 in different states of India is given in figure 4. The maximum increase in number of pigs was in the state of Tripura (+37.48%) and maximum decrease in number of pigs was in the state of Odisha (-54.17).

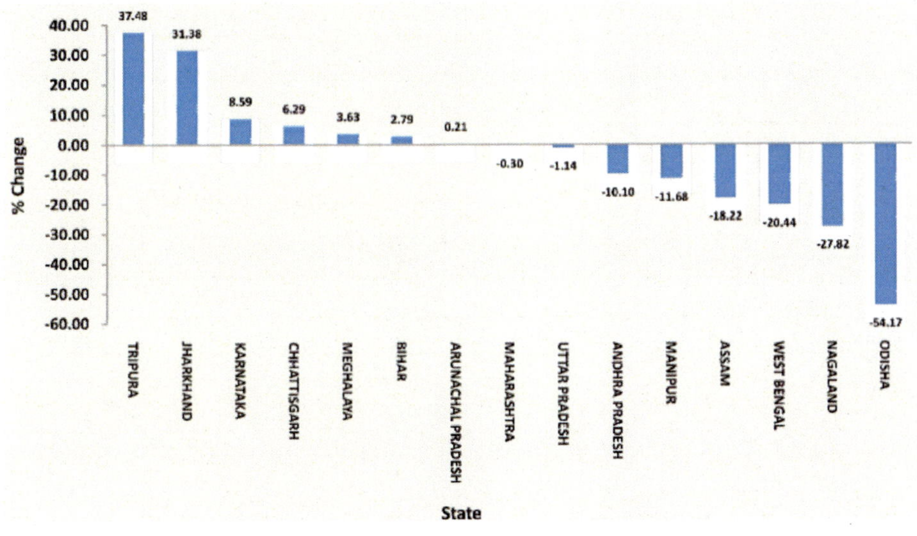

Fig. 4. Percent change in the population of pigs from 2007 to 2012 in different states of India
(*Source:* 19th Livestock Census-2012, Government of India)

Excessive slaughter to meet the demand of pork and destruction of a large number of pigs due to zoonotic diseases which had a sudden, and large incidence in the last few years. There are large socio-economic and socio-cultural differences and most large communities and larger part of the country do not like to rear pigs or consume pork. There was a continuous rise in population from 1951 to 1966 though at a slow rate and from 1966 to 2003 relatively rapid and this was followed by a steep decline. The population grew by 32.7% from 1961 to 71. However subsequently it declined from 2003 to 2012. The challenge before the R&D organizations is to reverse the declining trend through proper control of mortality and eradication of the zoonotic diseases which affect pigs and have resulted in their large scale destruction, rather than an increasing demand for pork and pork products in the traditionally high consuming regions such as North-East as well as in most large urban areas. Since pig has a high prolificacy and survival, it is easier to increase their numbers. Use of AI can help in propagation of exotic/superior indigenous breeds and their crosses with indigenous breeds/types.

Although the pigs are distributed throughout the country especially in the rural and peri-urban areas, the North-Eastern states due to largest consumption of pork have small population ranging from 3 to 5% of the total country's population. The growth rate in pig population during 2003-12 has been 19% in rural areas and 49% in urban areas.

Requirement and production of pork has been worked out and according to Indian Council of Medical Research (ICMR) an adult Indian should consume 60g protein daily of which 1/3 (20g) should be of animal origin. Considering that 50% of the population is non-vegetarian and of that 20% consume pork i.e. 10% of the total population obtains their animal protein from pork, the total requirement would be 0.44 m indicating a shortage of 0.11m or 25%. Globally the pork constitutes 36% followed by poultry (mostly chicken) 35%, beef and kine (buffalo meat) 27%, mutton and chevon 4.6%. In India, beef and kine constitutes 42%, followed by poultry 36%, mutton and chevon 14% and pork 5%. India exports a small quantity of pork but imports pork products especially bacon and sausages.

Inspite that there is a sharp growing demand for non-vegetarian food, for large urban population, it consumes a large part of processed food of which meat is a large component. There is a possibility of an increase in consumption of pork and pork products. Pig being a non-ruminant would compete not only with chicken but also with man for grain and soya products. Further the pig has an important public health implication, because of zoonotic disease like Classical Swine Fever, Porcine Reproductive and Respiratory Syndrome, Porcine Rotavirus and Paro virus infection. The way pigs are maintained under more extensive management with little surveillance and monitoring and prophylactic measures, the increase in pig production especially in peri-urban and urban areas can cause serious health problems, if proper measures for containment of pig diseases of zoonotic significance are not taken.

The decadal growth in population and pork production was 3.4 percent against the world of 5.00 and 15.45 percent. Neither the population nor the productivity of pork has been rising and the current R&D programs are making little impact on pig production in the country. There is a need to investigate the reasons. One of the possible reason can be destruction of a large population of pigs due to emerging diseases of zoonotic importance, necessitating elimination of a large proportion of pig population.

The SWOT (Strengths, Weakness, Opportunities, and Threats) analysis of pig sector indicates that with a population of 10.29 m in 2014, it is not able to provide the requisite proportion of animal protein which would be available from of all domestic animals. Pigs are able to perform more efficiently even under relatively low production inputs and poor management conditions. Pigs can, therefore; be reared by economically, socially and culturally deprived classes of people as the indigenous pigs do not require any production and protection inputs in terms of supplementary feed to what is naturally available from scavenging, protection from inclement weather through housing, protection from common diseases through vaccination and internal and external parasitic control and can be marketed readily. It is easier to increase or decrease the strength of a herd because of high reproduction rate and large demand of live animals for slaughter. Pig by-products especially bristles and non-edible offal are able to support rural industries. Both commercialization and organic pork production are strengths for increasing pig production. The Government of India and State Governments are promoting pig production through various poverty alleviation and employment generation programs and are providing large grants and loans at low rate of interest. Pork is a popular meat among economically and socially poor people and among neo-rich urban population and there is a growing demand for raw pork and processed products. Promoting pig production programs can help in poverty alleviation and provision of high quality protein food to rural and peri-urban poor and some income to meet the expenditure on other household needs.

Pig production, however, is not popular in a large part of the country and among economically and socially better of people because of religious taboo and pig being considered essentially a dirty animal because it consumes all human waste and can transmit zoonotic diseases. There is no regulated pig market where live animals can be sold. Pigs are purchased by the meat shops as and when there is a demand for meat. There is a large preference of meat of indigenous pigs which are relatively inefficient in pork production because of poor reproduction rate, live weight gain, efficiency of feed conversion, carcass yield and quality. The non-availability of adequate numbers of improved piglets either indigenous or crosses with exotic breeds, cheap feed and adequate health and marketing facility are constraints in intensifying pig production. Pig is an efficient converter of low quality feed, collected through scavenging or collected by owner from restaurants, eateries, vegetable and fruit markets / processing facilities, slaughterhouse, which; if properly processed and fed to pigs, can improve their production and make pork production more competitive. Pig production is generally associated with socially and economically backward people and there are a large number of programs to technically and financially assist them. Pig production requires low investment, has faster turnover, can be an attractive possibility in poverty alleviation and food and nutritional security enhancement programs. Since pigs have a higher reproduction rate, the pig keepers can be encouraged not only to raise pigs to be marketed for slaughter but to establish other units which will have a multiplier effect. Organizing pig producers into a cooperative or a producer company for establishing a pig breeding farm to provide young piglets to the members of the cooperative or producer group and help in collective provision of other inputs and services such as feed collected from hotels and eateries, fruit and vegetable markets, fruit processing units etc. and bulk process such feed and make it available to pig producers. They can also be helped in processing and marketing of meat and other byproducts such as bristles which can be used for making brushes and thus provide an additional self employment and income opportunity. Establishment of a processing unit for making value added products with longer shelf life and higher consumer acceptability can help in further improving the economics of pig production.

1.6 Strategies for developing pig production in lower resources endowed areas and by economically and socially deprived communities

Feeding strategies: Identification of cheap feed resources such as agro-industrial processing by-products, cheaper sources of energy such as broken grains and coarse grains, cheaper oil cakes / meals, roots such as sweet potato, cassava, food and fruit processing wastes, hotel wastes can help in meeting the nutritional requirements at a relatively lower cost compared to intensive feeding on feed grains and oilcakes. Meat meal and fish meal can provide excellent source of protein with essential amino acids. The provision of adequate housing space and comfort by keeping the pig sties clean and dry, protection of piglets being crushed by their mother and timely protection against infectious diseases and internal and external parasites and provision of supplementary iron to piglets to avoid piglet anemia, are important procedures that should be followed for economic pig production.

There is a need to identify specific factors which will sustain production under available management inputs and ensure their proper exploitation for identified economic traits which improve productivity and marketability under the prevailing condition in specific agro-ecological, socio-economic and cultural conditions.

There is a need to ensure that the available genetic resources are systematically surveyed, conserved and utilized. Institutional support should be provided both in terms of finances as well as production inputs and services to ensure viable pig production enterprise.

Possible opportunities for facilitating pig production under poverty alleviation programs

i) This may involve adoption of improved pig production practices.

ii) Women empowerment through employment and increased income through pig production.

iii) Developing pig producers cooperatives or producer companies for collective provision of inputs and services for production, protection and processing and marketing of pigs and collective insurance and obtaining institutional financial support from the development agencies / banks. These may involve 10-20 pig producers per group and these groups can be further unionized at district level or federated at state level.

iv) The State Development Agencies and R&D organizations should help in identifying technologies which are acceptable to the pig producers in transforming pig production according to their need and socio-economic conditions.

v) Creation of piglet producing units so that the piglets are easily available to the cooperative producers.

vi) Provide production and health inputs collectively so that the delivery system is more effective, both in terms of reach and cost.

vii) Training of pig producers in improved management practices and collectively producing, processing and marketing through procurement and provision of inputs and services and also take collective processing and marketing of live animals and meat.

viii) Collective insurance against mortality.

ix) Institution of genetic improvement program through provision of AI services with genetically superior boars of the indigenous/exotic breeds/ their crosses.

x) Formulation of pig development strategies to ensure better self employment, incomes and thus poverty alleviation.

xi) Establishment of collective pig slaughter, meat processing, and marketing facilities.

xii) Ensuring proper sanitary and zoo-sanitary conditions.

xiii) Establishment of collective nucleus breeding farm for undertaking selection and as producing genetically superior males for use in the herds of cooperative pig producers.

Such interventions can improve sustainability of pig production system through

i) Nutrient recycling such as through feeding crop by-products, food processing industries by-products, hotel and restaurant leftover food, cultivated root crops such as cassava, sweet potato.

ii) Providing supplementary feed to scavenging pigs and intensive feeding of genetically selected or improved pigs through crossbreeding and proper processing and marketing of live pigs / pig products.

iii) Keeping a range of DAs including pigs so that the waste of one species can meet the feed needs of the other species.

iv) Pest and disease control, management, economic considerations, especially risk, prevention and ready cash flow can help in providing greater stability to a pig enterprise.

v) Integrating pig farming with other crop and or DA/ fish farming systems can help reducing economic perturbation at household level during physical or social stressful circumstances, the use of DAs waste as fertilizer, fuel and for generating food and cash through sale, can help in better economic maintenance of the families of DA keeper

vi) Utilizing pig manure for improving soil structure and fertility.

vii) Increasing economic efficiency through determining the size of the pig unit and integrating piggery with other DAs, crop and fish production. Integrated farming system allows recycling of the waste of one component as a feed stock for the other.

viii) In addition to enhancing production / productivity, attention should also be given to quality of produce and market acceptability and this should have least environmental negative effects.

❑❑❑

CHAPTER-2

Indigenous and Exotic Pig Genetic Resources - Need for Proper Description, Evaluation, Sustainable use and Conservation

The Indian wild pig (*Sus scrofa cristatus),* is still found in the Siwaliks and the Tarai area throughout Northern India. It lives on tall grasses, insects and offal of dead animals and discarded parts of slaughtered / game animals. The male is aggressive and even attacks human beings. All domesticated types except the Chinese type have descended from the Indian wild pig. The pig breeding originated in India and east Turkistan and spread through the Mediterranean region to Europe. The Chinese type is the descendent of *Sus vittatus* found wild in South East Asia. The European pigs are the descendent of the wild pig (*Sus scrofa). Sus scrofa and Sus vittatus* are connected by transitional races found in the geographical intermediate areas. The Mediterranean races are intermediate between the European and Eastern Asiatic types in several aspects. It seems that the domesticated pig was repeatedly made independently from the wild type all over the world where it is found.

The remains of pigs were found in Mohenjo-Daro and were present in large numbers from the very earlier times of their evolution when Mohenjo-Daro was a flourishing city. But it appears impossible to determine whether or not the pig was actually domesticated in this region or even whether it was used as a source of food by the inhabitants in those far of times. At present, the pigs are commonly found throughout these parts of the country and it is possible that during the ancient times they existed in large herds which roamed the countryside in search of food.

During the Neolithic period while people were hunting wild animals and subsisting on their meat and fruits of the wild jungle trees, a remarkable development took place in Western Asia that is the discovery of agriculture. It is the animals that live in herds / flocks, are easier to be domesticated. The herd / flock is generally led by a leader, generally the leader is a strong male whom the herd / flock follows and if the leader is captured the whole herd can easily be captured. Sheep, goats, cattle and pigs which are the main domesticated animal species come under this category. Similarly among the plants, it is the grasses, which tend to grow densely and are most amenable to be controlled by man. Most of the cereals of modern day world viz. wheat, barley, oats, and rice are essentially grasses.

The domestication of animals is closely related to sedentarization of human population and initiation of agriculture. The fact is proved by archeological excavations which show that animal husbandry and agriculture developed simultaneously. The large ruminants viz. cattle and buffaloes possibly came as crop robbers to the fields created by human civilization of Sindh and Punjab in the pre Harappans period. They were captured by the farmers and were domesticated. The pig is also a crop robber and even now wild pig is a pest in sugarcane and other root crop fields. There is a close relationship between the vegetation, animals and man. Domesticated animals provide man with food in the form of meat and milk, and draught animal power for crop production and transport of man and materials.

2.1 Indigenous pig genetic resources

Although no serious efforts for identification, description and evaluation of pig genetic resources in India has been made, a large number of genetic variants / breeds have been identified and described on the basis of their physical conformation, with a little emphasis on production and adaptation characters. These are essentially available in different regions and states of the country and have accordingly been named. These are Ankamali found in Kerala, Tamil Nadu, Karnataka and Maharashtra; Andaman wild pig found in Andaman island, Ghungroo found in West Bengal, Nicobari found in Nicobar island, Mali found in Tripura, Khasi local found in Meghalaya, Dome found in Tripura, Manipur Desi found in Manipur, Suwo found in Nagaland, Zovawk found in Mizoram, Lapcha Moun found in Sikkim, Doom found in Assam, Burdi found in Odisha, Pondi / Jhinga and

Golla found in Odisha. NBAGR through its network projects implemented in collaboration with SAUs / SVUs and some other agencies has taken up description and some evaluation of indigenous breeds of pigs in the countries both at physical and molecular level.

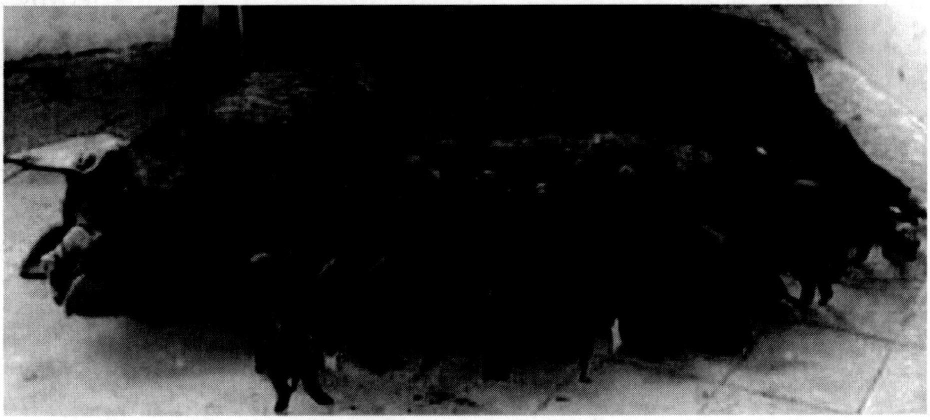

Ghungroo (*Source:* icar.org.in)

Little efforts have been made so far for fuller description and evaluation of these types / breeds, what to say for their sustainable management and conservation. Efforts are now being made by the NRC Pig and AICRP units of Pig for identification, description and evaluation of the different breeds in their respective regions and take steps for their sustainable management and conservation. The indigenous breeds in any region are generally smaller in size with hairy and black coat color and elongated face with long snout and short ears. They have early sexual maturity, shorter inter-farrowing interval and have reasonably large litter size. Most of the pig types in North-East have been named after the tribe which rears them or the area in which they are reared. Some of the breeds / types are available in more than one location such as Doom is found in Assam and Meghalaya, similarly Naga local are found in Nagaland, Mizo / Zovawk in Mizoram and Mali in Tripura. Physical conformation of some of the breeds has been described by Assam Agricultural University, ICAR Research Complex for NEH region and NRC Pig. Scavenging system and backyard rearing are most common management systems. Scavenging system is more common in Assam where the pigs are let loose for scavenging during the day and are sheltered during night. Backyard rearing system is most common in tribal belt of NE region. The pigs are kept in temporary shelters constructed with locally available material mostly wood logs and bamboos and are protected from rains and snow with a tin roof. The pigs are generally maintained in the backyard for easy handling and feeding on household waste.

2.1.1 Naga local

Pigs are generally pygmy or miniature in size and were essentially wild till they were domesticated more recently. They are generally reared in backyard. They are black in color with black or black diamond or star shaped white patches on the forehead. White hair below the foot lock and hock joint and on belly line in ventral surface and on the switch of the tail which is generally white, are the major characteristics of the breed. They are very active and alert. The skin is smooth and white to grey in color. They are uniformly covered with black hair and the mid line has moderate bristles. The ears are small and erect. The females are pot bellied but ventral line is straight in males, the teats are needle type and number 4-5 pairs. These pigs have long straight snout which is pointed and white in color with highly tapering nostrils. They have medium sized tail. The puberty is reached at around two months and the animals can be impregnated as early as five months. The birth weight of male piglet ranges between 300-500 gm and reaches 2.5 to 3.0 kg at three months of age. Puberty is attained at 90 days when the animal attains 3 kg live weight. Tabieu and Meishan breeds of china also attain puberty at 90 days of age but have higher live weight at puberty (20 Kg) compared to only 3 kg of Naga local pigs. Under traditional production management, the males attain adult live weight of 30-40 kg and females 25-38 kg. However, under intensive feeding and better management, the males can attain 38.9±2.8 kg and females 34.5±1.3 kg adult live weight.

2.1.2 Burmese pigs

Are found in Mizoram and Nagaland adjoining Burma (Myanmar). The animals are long and have arch shaped back in males. They resemble large black Ghungroo pigs. The head is broad with short and curved snout, undulated drooping ears which nearly cover the eyes in adults affecting their vision. The animals are docile, have good litter size at birth and weaning.

2.1.3 Zovawk pig of Mizoram

Which means Mizo pig. It has a small size. The population is declining. The animals are found in isolated pockets. They are predominantly black in color with white spot on forehead and white boots. The adult males are pot bellied with drooping backline. Birth weight averages 0.2 kg in males and 0.49 kg in females and weaning weight averages 4.7 kg in males and 3.61 kg in females. Average Daily Gain (ADG) in males averages 66 gm and in females 64 gm.

2.1.4 Mizo local pigs

Are small in size, pot bellied, hairy, and black in color with elongated face and short ears. These are early maturing and farrow early for the first time. The average weight at 9 months is 30.9 kg. They are inferior in performance than their crosses with exotic breeds.

2.1.5 Khasi local / Meghalaya local

Are mostly black in color with diamond or star shaped white marking on the forehead. The legs below the hocks are white. The animals have wild look, have smaller and stronger forelegs. Ears are small and erect. The belly almost touches the ground. The age at first farrowing averages 33 days with inter-farrowing interval of 210 days, weaning weight averages 5 kg.

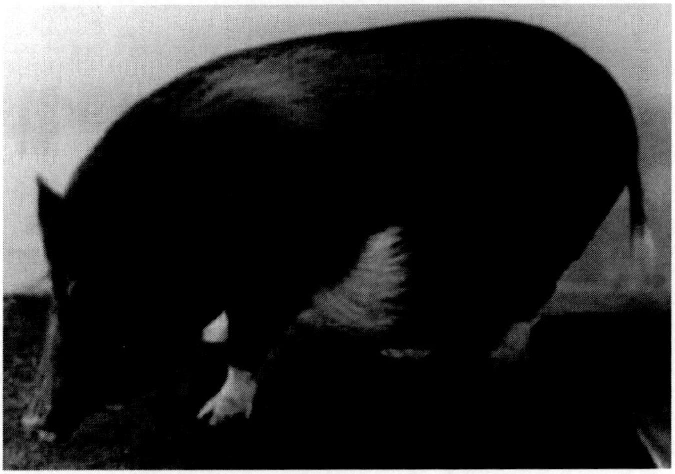

Niang Megha (*Source:* icar.org.in)

2.1.6 Mali pigs

Are black in color with compact body, thick coarse long hair, short legs and long tail. The face is narrow with upwardly curved snout. Ears are erect. Hind quarters are medium in size and rump is looping. Males are aggressive and females show strong mothering ability, nesting / burrowing is common in sows under rural conditions. They are ferocious immediately before and after farrowing. Males attain puberty at 138 days and females at 118 days. Gilts are bred at second and third heat. Estrous cycle is of 21 days, gestation period and farrowing interval averages 115 and 178 days respectively. Average litter size at birth is 8.6 and is 7.5 at weaning. Body weight at birth, weaning, 5 months, 1 year average 65 g, 4 kg, 27 kg, and 71 kg respectively. The average age at first farrowing is 281 days. Soon after weaning sows come in heat. Pre-weaning mortality averages 13%. The animals reach market weight of 70 kg in 1-1.5 years of age.

2.1.7 Nicobari pig

Nicobari pig is short, black and brownish in color. The coat color is black. The ears are straight and 6 inch long and 4 inch wide. The color is grayish white. The hoof color is also grayish white. The body length and chest girth in males average 43 and 33 inches. The height averages 23 inches.

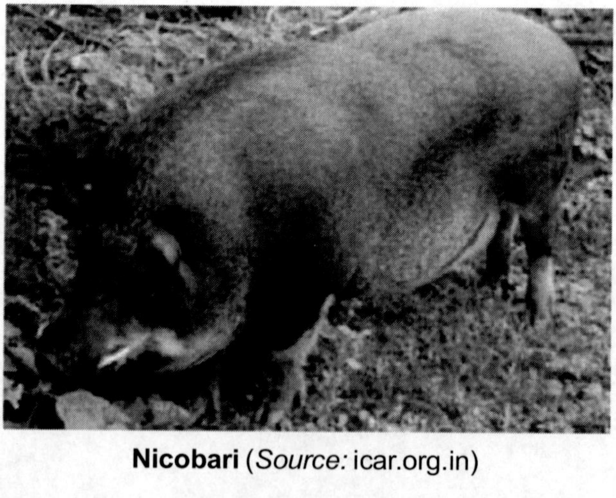

Nicobari (*Source:* icar.org.in)

2.2 Exotic breeds of pigs imported in India and used as purebreds or in grading local descript / non-descript pigs

2.2.1 Large white / Yorkshire

The breed was developed in England and became also popular in Northern Ireland. The breed is white in color on entire body, has slightly dished face, leveled back, fine pink skin with wrinkles and long deep sides, and long thin and projecting head. The breed is valued for bacon production. It is rugged and hardy breed and can stand wide variations in environment effects. The breed has been used for making improvement in other exotic breeds for bacon and pork quality. The adult weight ranges from 300-400 kg in males and 230-320 kg in females. They produce large litter at farrowing and weaning because of heavy milk production and excellent maternal instinct. Their extra height or length of leg helps them to remain active. They have long productive life. The breed is often used in rotational crossing using two or more breeds for efficient pork production.

2.2.2 Large Black also known as Cornwall, Devon, Lopeared Black

It was developed as black pig of Devon and Cornwall and these pigs are found in East Anglia. It became a well known breed after 1900. It is only slightly smaller than Yorkshire. It has long head, straight face with loop ears, a deep body, fair length and strong peck. The breed has fine hair with thick black pigment. The ears are so long they can cover most of the face and obstruct the vision. The breed is very docile and is resistant to major diseases and produces quality meat efficiently. Because of large litter size and good mothering ability, it is used as dam breed in crossing for commercial pig production.

2.2.3 Tamworth

This is a superior breed and is most active of the exotic pig breeds, is highly pre-potent and leaves the mark on the breed it is crossed with. The breed originated in Ireland and also called Irish grazer. The coat color is generally red but may vary in intensity from golden to dark red. The breed is deep sided with uniform depth, has arched back and a muscular but has relatively narrow back and a long rump. The ham produced is muscular and firm. The breed has long neck, long legs but lacks width. It has fine trimmed jowl, firm underline and firm fleshing. It has a striking head, i.e. long with a moderately long snout which is quiet straight. The breed has been evolved through long term selection for meat quality to make most desirable bacon. The breed is rugged, thrifty and very active. It produces lean meat. The sows are excellent mothers and can raise large litters.

2.2.4 Berkshire

The breed has originated in Thames valley around 1790 AD and was responsible for bringing improvement in pig production in USA and most of Europe. The breed has been improved by its association which is 100 years old. The breed has played an important role in pig industry. The meat is fine textured and has distinct flavor. The carcass weight ranges from from 36-45 kg. The breed can be used as sire and dam line and when mated to white colored breeds produce white colored progenies. It can withstand extremes of temperature. It has excellent carcass quality.

2.2.5 Hampshire

It is one of the oldest breed of the pigs in the world and has been evolved in North America. It probably originated from an old British breed. It is black in color with a white belt around the body. It is medium in size with male weighing between 250-350 kg and sows between 200-300 kg. Piglets weigh 1.2-1.5 kg at birth. The breed has good foraging habit.

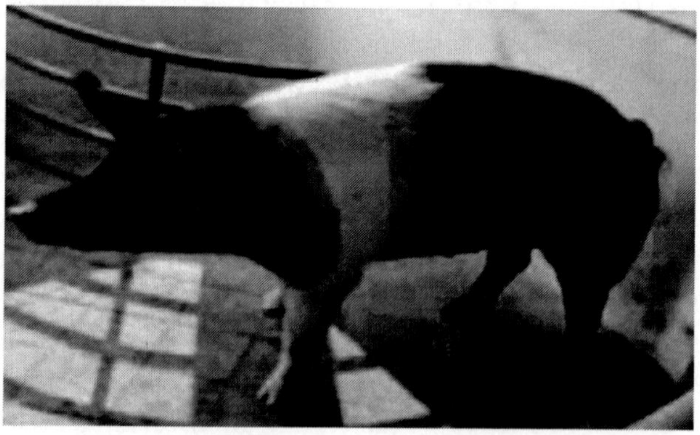

Hampshire (*Source:* icar.org.in)

2.2.6 Duroc

The breed had originated in eastern USA which is the corn growing belt. It is large bodied, late maturing with heavy carcass yield. The head and neck are light, ears are small and lop shaped, and the color is solid red varying from golden to deep brick red. It has medium length and slightly dished face. It is a small sized breed and more compact than other European breeds and produces quality meat at an early age. Duroc is generally used as a terminal sire breed on a two breed cross. The Duroc and Duroc crosses make good maternal sire line. The litter size is relatively lower than other European breeds.

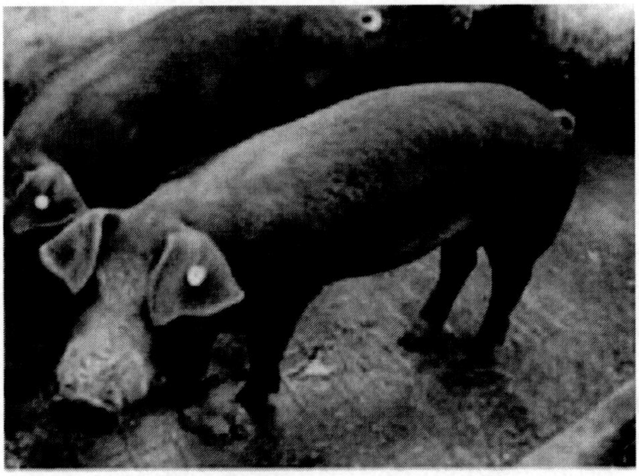

Duroc (*Source:* kiran.nic.in)

2.2.7 Landrace

The breed was developed in Denmark by crossing the local pigs with Large White. The crosses were interbred and improved through selection. The breed is white in color, heavy drooping ears that cover much of the face, has very long muscular body and produces high quality pork. The breed has white skin and is free from black hair. The breed produces excellent ham. It is highly prolific and is docile breed. The breed is used for crossing with other European breeds for producing quality bacon.

2.3 Genetic improvement

Genetic improvement in productivity involves appropriate selection and mating systems

The breeding strategies for improving pig production would require definition of breeding goals, identifying breed / breeds, select male and female parents, decision on appropriate mating plan suitable to meet the production goals and the economic conditions in which the production is aimed at.

2.3.1 Selection

Important economic traits in improving pig production are birth weight, weaning weight, litter size at birth and weaning, litter weight at birth and weaning, individual piglet weight at 60 days, 90 days and 180 days. The reproduction traits of interest are age at first oestrus, oestrous cycle length, age at first service, age at first fertile service, age at first farrowing, gestation length, service period and inter - farrowing interval. The carcass traits of interest are carcass length, dressed weight and dressing percentage, loin eye area, percentage primal cuts and meat: bone ratio.

Genetic improvement through selection would depend on heritability of individual economic traits of interest, whether they are sex linked or sex limited, qualitative/quantitative in measurement. The selection may be based directly on traits of interest or on correlated traits. Selection method may be random selection, independent culling levels for each trait in a sequences or index selection. Further selection may be based on individual performance, pedigree, collateral relatives such as paternal/maternal half sibs or full sibs or progeny. The selection will be based on individual performance, pedigree performance, and family performance such as collateral relatives or on progeny performance.

Genetic progress through selection would depend on selected high performing stocks, prolificacy, growth rate, temperament, carcass yield and quality, efficiency of feed conversion, combining ability in case of more than one breed is involved, market demand for the produce and disease resistance. The breeders may be selected on the basis of litter size and weight, body weight gains up to six months of age or for the market weight desired, efficiency of feed conversion, longevity, fertility, and freedom from any physical defects.

The boar may be selected on its conformation to the breed type, muscular appearance, long deep body, strong legs and smooth shoulders, sound health and good performance record for various production traits related to reproduction, live weight gains, dressing percentage, carcass yield and meat quality in progeny, and longevity. The animals should not be cryptorchid, should be tested for fertility such as libido, semen quality, and fertilizing capacity. The animal should have good physical appearance, strong back, and active appearance. The sows should be from a large litter at birth and weaning, should have at least 6 pairs of teats evenly distributed and have minimum back fat thickness. The teats should be free from any abnormality. It should have deep body, should preferably once earlier farrowed and must be two to three year old, should have high milk production and strong mothering ability. Inspite all these traits are of economic importance but since they express and a few of them express in either sex or late in life or require slaughter, it is desirable that few of the traits which are expressed early in life and explain a large percentage of variation in traits expressed late in life or are limited to one sex or need slaughter can help in increasing genetic progress in overall merit of a selected animal.

The breeding systems may involve inbreeding to increase homozygosity, develop inbred lines to increase purity of a breed and eliminate undesirable recessive genes. Inbreeding generally leads to reduction in reproductive efficiency, growth rate, milk production and mothering ability, and increases mortality and morbidity, sex libido in males and fecundity and prolificacy in females. However, inbreeding is essential to remove undesirable recessive alleles and to create pure lines which when crossed would provide maximum heterosis and thus improves survival and growth. In pigs generally two way or three way crosses are practiced. Initially lines selected for body weight gains and carcass (meat) quality characteristics in one line, fertility and young survival in the other line are selected or crossed and the crosses are bred with a breed with high carcass yield and quality as a terminal breed which is used on two way cross female. All the progeny of the terminal mating are disposed of and are not used for further breeding.

Genomic research in pig

Pig genomic sequence is not only important for revealing the present characters related to production, reproduction and adaptation, but also understanding the evolution and subsequent (genetic) changes that have resulted in the present genetic structure and the variability in a population. Pig has served as a model for behavioral and disease studies in human. Pig is being modified to develop its organs for transplantation in human beings, it is also being used as model for studies on human diseases like obesity, arthritis, cardio-vascular diseases, etc. It is also being used as a biomedical model and could serve as a template for the study of within and between species genetic variation. The pig has 18 pairs of autosomes and one pair of sex chromosome being XX and XY. It is similar to size (2.7×10^9 bp) complexity of chromosomal organization including meta-and acrocentric chromosomes which are similar to the human genome, comparative genetic merits indicates that the porcine and human genome are more similarly organized than when compared to mouse, the mean length of conserved syntenic segments between human and pig genomes is approximately twice as long as the average length of conserved syntanic segments between human and mouse. Further the organizational similarities between the genomes of the two species reflect of the same at nucleotide levels.

Genetic research in pigs so far has been mostly related to improvement of quantitative (genetic) traits since most of the traits of economic importance in the pigs are polygenic in nature and with appropriate use of quantitative genetic techniques, the knowledge provided has given an opportunity for maping a growing number of QTLs, the first linkage map was published in 1994 and has been used in identifying chromosomal regions associated with quantitative traits like growth, carcass composition, reproduction and immune response. Similarly cDNA libraries have been developed at different physiological stages for many different traits and more than 100,000 expressed tags (ESTs) have been deposited at the Institute of Genetic Research. EST mapping is improving human-pig comparative maps. The TIGR cluster analysis on EST sequences has generated more than 50,000 non-redundant gene indices that are routinely used by the International Genetic Research Community. Based on human genomic sequences, a subset of 1000 ESTs has been selected for sequencing predicted introns to indentify SNP for mapping of linkage map. The porcine genome RH map integrates micro-satellite markets and ESTs BLAST fix with human sequences. This map contains more than 5,500 STS markers and is being assembled with more than 2,000 comparative markers. An international consortium has been set up to construct the porcine bacterial artificial chromosome (BAC) map which includes INRA in France, Roseline in U.K., Sanger Institute, University of Illinois and OIS and USDA-ARS in U.S.A.

Two methods namely linkage and linkage disequilibrium analysis have been utilized to map QTL. Most QTL studies using families derived from divergent crosses and low resolution maps used linkage analysis to localize specific traits to chromosomal regions of less than 10 cM have been made. On the other hand LD is highly informative but is dependent upon a high resolution map of both existing populations and family data can be incorporated and high density SNP maps prepared to provide a powerful approach for multi-point fine mapping and traits difficult to map such as disease resistance. More recently regression approach for mapping QTL by LD using population data has been achieved with complex trait with 250 sample size with moderate LD. This proves the high utility of LD for mapping QTL and most QTL studies are limited in the number of phenotypic scores. LD is also referred to as allelic associate and with the development of SNP based LD maps for genome association studies, it would be possible to have a more efficient detection of candidate disease resistance or susceptibility genes.

2.4 Research initiatives in improving pig production

Programmes for improving pig production have been undertaken by the Central and State Governments since independence but the major initiatives came in 4th five year plan when the ICAR initiated an AICRP on pigs with the objectives of studying the performance of pure bred exotic breeds. The breeds involved were Landrace and Large White Yorkshire. Centers were located at ANGRAU Tirupati, AAU, Khanapara and JNKVB, Jabalpur and IVRI, Izatnagar. The coordinating unit and a germplasm center was located at IVRI. Subsequently, Tamilnadu University of Veterinary and Animal Sciences (TANUVAS) and Kerala Agricultural University (KAU), Mannuthy were included. The ICAR Research Complex Goa Center, Birsa Agricultural University (BAU), Ranchi were added in 2000-01 and Central Agricultural University, Izol campus, and Nagaland University were included but JNKVB, Jabalpur unit was discontinued.

During the 4th and 5th five year plan, the project envisaged to study purebred performance of the two exotic breeds viz., Large White Yorkshire at Tirupati and Jabalpur and Landrace at Khanapara and Izatnagar. The project envisaged (i) to asses various genetic parameters of economically important traits related to production, reproduction and efficiency of feed utilization, (ii) to investigate the effect of protein: energy and evolve a low cost/ economic ration and (iii) to study disease incidence and devise suitable control measures.

At the end of 6th plan, it was decided that in the light of larger population of pigs being non-descript and relatively low producing and maintained under scavenging and with little supplementary feed input. These pigs not only have a large population and spread but are of high economic importance to the rural poor. The technical programme was subsequently modified to include crossbreeding with appropriate exotic breeds in addition to studies on performance of indigenous types of pigs under optimum management, undertake crossbreeding of indigenous with exotic breeds and assess the performance in terms of live weight gains efficiency of feed conversion, carcass yield and quality, reproduction. The project also emphasized on evolving economic pig ration from locally available conventional and non-conventional feed resources. The halfbreds were to be selected for growth rate using economic ration and study incidence of various diseases and effective prophylactic measures.

Subsequently, the programme was changed during the 10th plan and envisaged that in light of small population size and selection being relatively ineffective, male should be replaced to more often to avoid inbreeding. Early weaning at 4 weeks of age should be practiced and piglets raised on nutritionally balanced creep feed. Region based shelter management and integrated farming systems such as crop and pigs and pig and fish should be studied for their economics. Efforts should be made to reduce overall mortality to less than 10% through forecasting disease incidence from meteorological factors and effective steps should be taken for the control of disease. Económic feed formulation based on the local resources should be developed but the feeding of the experimental stock should be on the laid down feed composition.

Subsequently a more detailed work plan for the existing and the new centers proposed to be included, was decided in 2013 and envisaged raising of animals with 75% exotic inheritance, their *inter se* mating and selection. It was envisaged that a minimum 30 breeding sows would be mated with 10 sires (3:1). The sires will arise from each five unrelated sires. The sires will be selected on the basis of an Index combining litter size at birth and weaning, litter weight at birth and weaning and the number of functional teats (a minimum of 6 pairs of functional teats). The selected animals would be further screened cytogenetically for detecting any genetic abnormality and if positive, would not be used for breeding. The selected males should have a live weight of 65 kg at 8 months. The litter size should be at least seven. The performance of the progeny should be studied in each generation to record the effectiveness of selection. AI should be introduced. The project also envisaged studies on nutrition, physiology, management and health to validate the existing feeding regime and evolve suitable location specific production technologies to reduce environmental stress based on temperature humidity index (THI). Infectious diseases should be properly recorded and their consequent mortality and morbidity should be studied.

The project has been able to develop methodology for (i) improving indigenous pigs through selection, (ii) studies on the performance of purebreds and crosses of Landrace and Large Yorkshire with indigenous types with 50% and 75% exotic inheritance and reciprocal crosses of those involving different breeds. It has been observed that exotic breeds of pigs viz Landrace Large, White Yorkshire can be raised successfully and bred under intensive farm management. Genetic improvement in indigenous pig can be brought through selection and /or crossbreeding with exotic breed. There is improvement in litter size at birth and weaning and live weight gains up to 32 weeks of age in crossbreds and purebreds. The selection within the indigenous pigs is slow, primarily due to small effective population size used and low intensity of selection, (iii) the crossbreds have bigger litter size, higher growth rate and better efficiency of feed conversion than the indigenous pigs, (iv) there was further improvement in litter size in increase exotic inheritance from 50 % to 75%. (v) Pig can be utilized effectively as a component of integrating farming system, and (vi) it was further observed that the crossbred involving exotic and indigenous breeds have lower back fat thickness and higher % of lean meat.

Studies on pig management have led to standardization of semen collection and AI technologies using liquid semen, development of automatic feeders, artificial milk feeding to orphaned piglets. Sprinklers for reducing heat stress and avoid wallowing, pressure cleaning system of pig sties and automatic waterers for pigs.

Nutritional studies have resulted in determining optimum energy and protein content in feed of different breeds and breed crosses and development of economic rations for different production types.

Studies on pig reproduction conducted have showed that the indigenous pigs both descript and non-descript have relatively lower litter size, live weights at different ages, live weight gains and efficiency of feed utilization but have higher lean meat. The crossbred with exotic breeds have improved litter size and survival, have better growth rate and efficiency of feed conversion than the indigenous pigs. The higher grades (75%) exotic inheritance have higher litter size than half breds.

In addition to the research initiatives under AICRP and now additionally at the NRC pigs, there have been initiatives of the different educational, research and development organizations. The initiatives of the TANUVAS on improving the profitability and resource use efficiency has shown that three way synthetic crossbreds involving Large White York Shire male and Land-race females and F1 females bred to Duroc males, resulted in a better performance in terms of body weight gains and carcass yield and quality. The three breed crosses had higher body weight by 4 kg that Large White York Shire at 8 weeks of age, higher efficiency of feed conversion, dressing percentage, lower back fat thickness and higher ham and bacon percentage.

Similarly in Kerala, Kerala Livestock Development Board (KLBD) is undertaking the sustainable management of local Angamaly pigs which are highly disease resistance, environmental stress resistance (temperature and humidity). Their crosses with exotic breeds such as Large White and superior indigenous breed have shown substantial improvement in overall performance. The KLDB is maintaining Large White Land Race and Duroc breeds and producing Large White x Land Race crossbred females and breeding them with Duroc to raise three breed crosses for fattening. Some exotic Asiatic breeds like Myanmar crossbred have been introduced to Manipur by indigenous pig breeders.

There are a large number of threats in the sustainable use and conservation in indigenous pig genetic resources, these are related to:

i) Unidentified and non-descript population which would require identification of all known and not known population, their description and evaluation through extensive surveys in their home tracts. The home tract will also have to be characterized in terms of topography, physical environment and vegetation resources. The population has to be characterized and documented and steps taken for the sustainable use and conservation/preservation depending upon the spread and the population size and structure including the current breeding programmes.

ii) The breeding strategy should be evolved to increase effective population size especially the number of sires used and their turn over, use in other population and change every third year, population trends, identify breeds under threat, establish nucleus population either on institutional farms with a representative sample or through an open nucleus involving a large number of herds with the pig keepers and undertaking intensive selection in the nucleus and supplying superior breeding males or their semen for AI. The use of advanced reproduction biotechnologies can help in increasing the population of breeds/types that are threatened to extinction.

iii) Improving the performance of the available breeds / strains through selection or grading with superior breed from comparable agro-ecology.

iv) Restricting excessive slaughter to maintain a large breeding population and using a relatively large number of breeding males and their faster turnover both for avoiding inbreeding and making faster genetic improvement.

v) Provision of adequate nutrition, health, management inputs and marketing facilities to sustain the existing production systems and bring further improvement.

2.5 Use of biotechnology in genetic improvement of pigs

2.5.1 Quantitative Trait Loci (QTL)

Crossing breeds for highly genetically divergent traits such as has been done using European wild bore on Large White. Within family linkage disequilibrium using large half sib families, there are a total of 9,862 QTLs for 653 different traits in pigs. After detecting the QTL, the gene responsive for the variation in the trait (causal mutation) needs to be identified. QTL is a region of about 20-40 cM, harboring some 200-400 genes. It is however difficult to identify the underlined genes responsible for the trait of interest especially with polygenic inheritance. Increasing the number of individuals, identifying their performance recorded and carry out their fine mapping or try the candidate gene approach. These approaches are currently difficult, expensive in recourses, and time, and have relatively lower success. Locating a gene responsible for the variation in an economic trait unless it has got a major effect is difficult. 9,000 QTCs have been reported in pigs of which less than a dozen causative mutations has been established.

2.5.2 Marker Assisted Selection (MAS)

It usually involves three steps (i) detection of one or several QTLs, (ii) the gene responsible for causal mutation and (iii) increasing of favorable allele either through selection or through introgression. MAS has been used successfully in genetic improvement of pigs through exploiting the existing genetic diversity in available populations and can be used to improve a range of desirable traits. DNA markers are polymorphic in nature and can be studied by restructured fragment length polymorphism (RFLPs), micro-satellite and single nucleotide polymorphism (SNPs), linkage analysis, associated analysis and analysis of gene function can be used to determine useful marker for the desired trait. Thus MAS can help in improving characters with low heritability those which are sex limited, express late in life, and require exposure to infection or needing slaughter. Within family linkage disequilibrium can be used in large half sib families within a breed. There are problems associated with false detection of related candidate genes. Using crosses between two breeds, a polymorphism on the estrogen receptor locus (ESR) has been associated to litter size in pigs within advantage of 1.5 piglets in homozygous sows for the beneficial allele. The effect of ESR gene varies widely among populations. The Table 1 gives genetic markers and the traits affected by them.

Table 1. Few examples of genetic markers and genes used in swine

Gene (action target)	Traits affected
RYR1 (halothane sensitivity)	Lean growth, porcine stress syndrome, meat quality
RN (Rendemement Napole)	Meat quality
ESR (estrogen receptor)	Litter size
PRLR (Prolactin receptor)	Nursing performance and litter size
RBP4 (retinol binding protein 4)	Litter size
MC4R (melanocortin-4 receptor)	Lean growth, fatness, feed intake
IGF2 (insulin-like growth factor 2)	Lean growth, litter size
HFABP/AFABP	Intramuscular fat
c-KIT receptor	Coat and skin colour
MC1R (melanocortin-1 receptor)	Red/ black coat colour
PRKAG3 (protein kinase AMP-activated gamma 3-regulatory subunit)	Meat quality
HMGA (high mobility group AT hook 1)	Backfat thickness
CCKAR (cholecystokinin type A receptor)	Feed intake and growth
CAST (Calpain inhibitor)	Tenderness
EPOR (erythropoietin)	Litter size
F18	Escherichia coli diarrhoea
K88	E.coli diarrhoea

2.5.3 Marker Assisted Introgression (MAI)

MAI involves identification of a desirable allele at a target locus from a donor breed and transfer it to a recipient breed through multiple back crossing and then one or more generation of interbreeding. The aim is to generate individuals that carry one copy of donor QTL allele. Marker information can enhance the effectiveness of back crossing for gene introgression through identifying carriers of the target gene (fore ground selection) and enhancing recovery of the recipient genetic back ground (back ground selection). Mostly MAI has involved single QTL but even several QTLs can be introgressed simultaneously. Large population size is required to obtain a sufficiently large number of individuals that are heterozygous for all QTLs in the back crossing phase. This would make MAI nor feasible in DA breeding programmes, now being implemented in DAs . If this objective is not important, back crossing can enrich with the favorable donor QTL alleles that can be selected on following back crossing.

2.5.4 Genomic Selection (GS)

This approach removes some of the limitations of MAS. The developments in genome sequencing, the identification of a large numbers of genetic markers across the genome in the form of SNPs on individual animals along with statistical methods for analysis of molecular data, genetic markers have been used for predicting breeding value for genomic selection (GS). The first step in GS is to collect phenotypic data and DNA from a large number of individual with phenotypic information or those with performance recorded on their progeny. Each animal is genotyped using SNP chip. The resulting data are being used in a statistical model that estimates the effect of each of the SNP on the SNP chip with the trait phenotype is employed. The resulting estimates can be used to predict genomic expected breeding value (EBV). GS has been used in pig breeding in accurately predicting breeding values in traits which otherwise will increase generation interval and controlling inbreeding. The effectiveness of GS depends on the level of linkage disequilibrium (LD) that can be utilized by markers within the target population.

2.5.5 Transgenic pigs

Altering genetic material to change the expression or increase the frequency of specific genes to ultimately result into a desired phenotype is transgenesis. The introduction of exogenous DNA through rDNA technology is the most common method, although the results can significantly vary and further depend upon whether the modification desired is random or specific. The use of lenti viruses has overcome limitations of viral mediated viral gene transfer which includes the silencing of the transgenic locus. With low expression levels. Injection of lenti viruses into the peri-viteline space of the porcine zygote has resulted in a high proportion of piglets carrying and expressing trans-gene. Stable transgenic lines have now been created.

2.5.6 Chimera generation via injection of pluripotent cells into blastocyst

ES cells with pluripotent characters can participate in organ and germ cell development after injection into blastocyst or by aggregation with morula. ES like cells and primordial germ cell have been cultured in several farm animal species and chimeric animals without germ line contribution have been developed. Somatic stem cells may have a much greater potential than the previously known.

2.5.7 RNA Interference

It is a conserved post-transcriptional gene regulatory mechanism in most biological systems. It includes siRNAs with 21 and 23 nucleotides which specifically bind complementary sequences on their target mRNAs and shut down their expression. The mRNAs are degraded by exo-nucleases and no protein is translated. It seems to be involved in gene regulation by controlling /and suppression of translation of mRNAs by endogenous viral elements. The mechanism has been adopted to generate transiently or permanently knocked down of specific gene.

2.6 Transgenic pigs for xeno-transplantation

For more than 50 years, pigs have been transformed for organ transplantation for humans as they have closer anatomical, physiological and genetic characters. A large number of genetic modifications such as adding complements modifies re-modeling the cell surface carbohydrates preventing anti-thrombosis and knocking out alpha -1,3-galactosyltrain transferase have been made to eliminate hyper-acute rejection and make the pig organ less immunogenic to the primates. The porcine endogenous retroviruses may impact transplantation but it is still not very clear. Knocking out of each retrovirus through cross genesis or through appropriate breeding strategies could remove retroviruses and make the pig organs fit for human transplantation. This is yet to be made possible.

2.7 Transgenic pigs for biomedical research

The pigs are more similar to human. Although the larger size of pig makes it more expensive as a model than smaller mammals and rodents, the size can be used with advantage for determining drug doses in pre-clinical trials and developing therapeutic strategies requiring surgical interventions. Transgenic pigs will continue to be used as models for human genetic studies such as muscular dystrophy, sickle cell anemia, genetic anomalies that cause a pre-disposition to specific cancer.

❑❑❑

CHAPTER-3

Pig Management

Pig is known to be a clean and efficient converter of feed both grains and agro-industrial processing by-products such as oilcakes/ meals, brans and polishes and also root crops such as cassava and beat root. However, majority of pig in India are maintained on free range scavenging with/without some supplementary feed based on house hold/market waste by-products. The age at maturity is low (4-5 months), gestation period is short (110-120) days, high prolificacy (8-12 piglets per farrowing) and at least two litters per year. In fact the management of reproduction is the key factor in maximizing pig production. In addition to young survival and growth, proper raising of piglets is important so that they can reach market weight early and thus save on the maintenance cost and can improve the economics of pig production.

Good management practices for improving pig production would involve:

i) Management of pregnant and farrowing sow
ii) Management of breedable males and females
iii) Rearing of piglets
iv) Nursery management to avoid being crushed by mother
v) Weather management to protect from inclement weather
vi) Housing
vii) Feed resource development and feeding
viii) Transport
ix) Disposal of animals and
x) Disease management

The care and management of gilts and sows during pregnancy is important to ensure proper health of the dams during pregnancy and pre-and post-farrowing period, growth and development of litter and ultimately litter size and litter weight which are also important for subsequent survival, growth and market weight. The gilts which do not show estrus within 21 days of service are normally considered pregnant. The date of service should be recorded so that she can be accommodated in a separate sty, measuring 3x2 meter, before farrowing. The floor of the farrowing pen should be clean, dry and should be non-slippery. The farrowing gilt/sow should be liberally fed at least 2-3 weeks prior to farrowing. This will help in improving weight and performing satisfactorily and post-natal survival and growth. They should be least disturbed a couple of weeks before farrowing and no abnormal behavior should be shown to them. They should not be walked long distance for feeding or watering. A bedding of 8-10cm in thickness of chopped straw should be provided. The animal should be separated 2-3 weeks before farrowing.

At the time of farrowing the care and management of sow should involve:

i) She should be washed and cleaned properly just before transfer to the farrowing pan.

ii) She should be transferred to the farrowing pen 8-10 days before farrowing to acclimatize her to the new environment.

iii) The farrowing pen should be provided with guard rails for protecting the piglets from being crushed by the sow when she lies down.

iv) The sow should be provided with bulky but highly digestive feed which should be reduced to the $1/3^{rd}$ till the time of the farrowing and withdrawn 12 hours before farrowing.

3.1 Care and management of post farrowing sow

i) Clean the hind quarters with warm water after farrowing.

ii) The piglets should be allowed to suckle the sow as soon as possible.

iii) If the milk of the dam is not being let down, oxytocin may be injected to help its letdown.

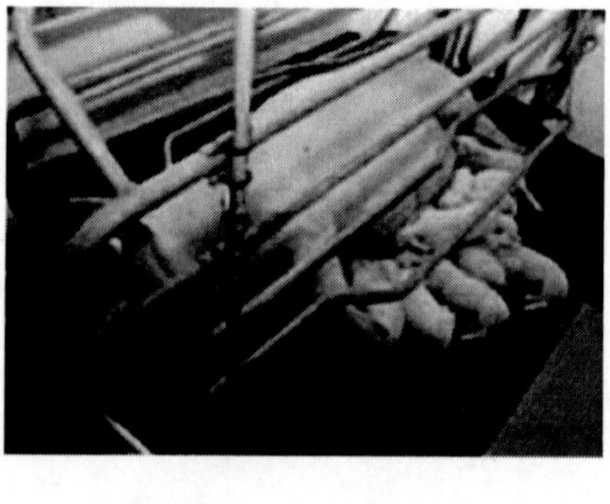

iv) Parturient sow should be provided first meal 12 hours after farrowing.

v) She should be provided clean and fresh water for drinking.

vi) The body temperature should be checked and if it is excessive high rectal temperature, appropriate treatment should be provided.

vii) Udder of the sow should be sprayed with saturated solution of iron sulphate to provide iron supplement and to prevent piglet anemia.

viii) Provide adequate balanced nutrient to the lactating sow to maximize milk production and proper rearing of piglets.

3.2 Management of breedable males and females

Selection of boars

A boar must conform to the breed type and must have high performance in terms of body weight gains and efficiency of feed conversion. It should come from a large litter weaned. The piglets to be used as boars should be selected between 20-30 weeks of age.

One boar should be allowed for 20 sows when hand mating is practiced. But under extensive management one boar should be allocated to 15-18 sows. The young boar should not be used for service until it is at least 28-30 weeks of age. Mating should preferably be carried out in the morning before feeding the animals. The number of services per conception would depend upon accurate detection of heat and proper timing of service. The service should be provided 12-18 hours after the detection of heat and repeated 12 hours later.

3.3 Care and management of piglets

i) An experienced person should be given charge to look after the farrowing sow and the new born piglets throughout the day and night.

ii) All breathing passages of piglets should be free from mucous. In case of difficulty in breathing, the piglets should be swung round at arm's length or immersed in cold water.

iii) The mucous should be removed from the body of the piglet and it should be dried with a clean cloth.

iv) Transfer piglets to a separate area with temperature ranging from 25-30 °C.

v) Prevent sow from eating her placenta and dispose of the placenta properly.

vi) Assist piglets to get to the teat and suckle the colostrum.

vii) The udder should be checked for agalactia (lack of milk), mastitis, number of teats to access its nourishing capacity in case the number of piglets is larger than the number of functional teats that the extra number of piglets should be artificially fed.

viii) The naval cord of the piglets should be cut with a sterilized knife and dressed with a disinfectant like tincture iodine/alcohol. In case of dystocia/difficult birth, proper assistance of qualified veterinarians should be provided. After farrowing in case of difficult birth, antibiotics may be administered to avoid metritis.

ix) Suitable micro-environment with proper light and heat should be provided especially during inclement weather to keep piglets comfortable.

x) Supplementary feeding of milk should be made available to piglets in case of inadequate mothering ability of the sow.

xi) The piglets should be identified by ear-notching or metal tagging in the ear. The former is a usual method for identification and is performed at one to two weeks of age. Hygienic measures and sterilization of the site of identification and notching equipment should be assured. While notching, the cutting of the ear vain should be avoided. The ear should be dressed with tincture of iodine after notching. Plastic tags are even better than metallic ear tags/notching as they can be read from a distance. For metal ear tagging, ear tagging machine is used. Tag with specified number, normally giving identification by farm, breed, sire and individual number is encrypted on the ear tag.

Administration of iron through injecting 0.5 ml of injectable iron irrespective of breed and the size of the animal on fourth and fourteenth day of age maintains the desired level of iron in the blood and prevents piglet anemia.

Male pigs not to be retained for breeding are generally castrated at a very young age and are put to fattening for the market. Castration removes undesirable breeding males and avoids indiscriminating mating. It also makes the males less aggressive and helps in producing superior quality pork with relatively less fat and prevents boar odor in the cooked meat. The castration should be done at three to four weeks of age. Open method of castration is generally used and it is desirable that the piglets should be kept off feed for 10 to 12 hours before open castration. The animal to be castrated should be properly secured by holding on dorsal side. The feet should be properly tied. A sterilized knife is used after cleaning the scrotum with an antiseptic solution and an incision is made on each side of the scrotum and the testis are removed with their membranes by pulling them backward and cutting the cord as high as possible. The scrotum is subsequently disinfected with tincture of iodine. No significant dressing is required.

Nursing of piglets

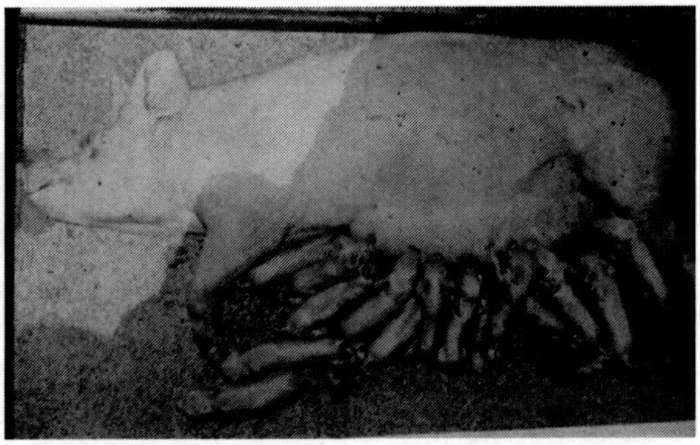

Piglets may be made to suckle within 6 hours of birth to consume colostrums. If they are unable to suckle or the mother is not responsive, the piglets should be helped to suckle. Colostrums prevents neonatal diseases by creating passive immunity, especially for the diseases the dam has been exposed to or vaccinated against them. If sufficient colostrum is not available, artificial milk feeding to the piglets should be resorted to. Early care and management of piglets is extremely important in ensuring their survival and early growth.

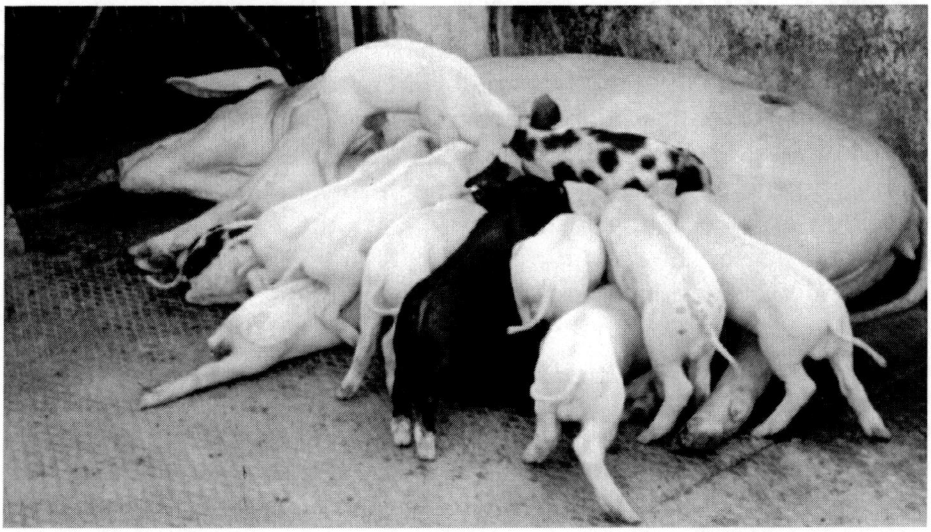

Weaning is generally done when the piglets have attained 4 to 5 kg. live weight or are around 30- 45 days of age . Weaning is highly stressful and affects piglet health and post weaning growth. Pre-weaning complications can be reduced by offering creep feeding from the age of 15 days.

3.4 Housing management

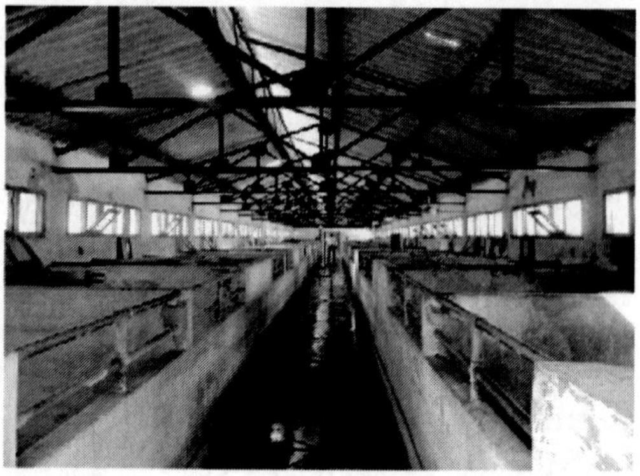

Except in highly intensive commercial pig farming involving genetically superior breeds specially exotic, pigs are generally kept in the open and allowed to fend for their feed from grasses, roots and insects but they should be protected from predation through keeping a proper watch. The ground where the pigs are maintained may be surrounded by a proper protecting fence made of thorny bushes or wire netting or a brick/mud wall. Since pigs have a habit of burrowing, proper flooring is desirable. Wooden or metal arks can be provided for the pigs to rest and should be covered with suitable bedding. The arks can be moved to fresh ground and the droppings removed and used as fertilizer. Generally bamboo and wooden material is used for making shelters, being cheap and easily available, and it is also easy to shift such shelters from one place to another. The floor should be raised above the ground level to avoid entry of reptiles, rats and other small wild predators. Such raised floors are also easy to clean and prevent dampening due to animal droppings and rain. The breeding sows and their litters can be maintained in sties or in the open fields with proper protection. It is desirable to provide proper bedding in the sty to keep the young piglets warm and comfortable. The bedding should be changed frequently. A railing is generally fixed along the wall so that the piglets can be prevented from being crushed when the lactating sows lies on top of them. Adult pigs can be kept in a group, in a sty which should be reasonably away from human dwellings to prevent menace of flies and bad smell. The floor should be of concrete, 5-6 cm thick and slopping from the wall where the animals tend to sleep. The walls of the sty should be fairly smooth as the cracks in the walls invite accumulation of dirt and breeding of insects. Proper bedding is helpful in keeping animals warm during winter and cool during summer and allows absorption of urine and thus keep the animal comfortable. However, the bedding should be changed as often as possible.

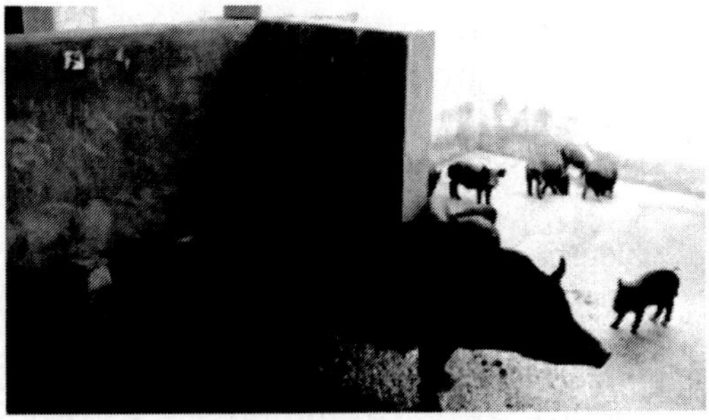

Guard-rail fitted half-walled sty with good ventilation and sunlight.

3.5 Feeding management

Pigs are omnivores and can consume both vegetable and animal origin feeds. Because of the structure of the mouth and teeth, the animals can consume plant materials from the ground. Being non-ruminant, they can utilize fibrous feeds only to a limited extent and that too less efficiently. Thus the feed must have more dense energy and protein to be consumed adequately to meet the maintenance and production requirements. Pig can utilize kitchen waste both from household and large eateries. It is a common practice to have disposal drums maintained at major hotels and restaurants or food processing units specially vegetable and fruits and the processing waste is collected, thoroughly mixed with other feed material specially cereal and oil seed processing byproducts and fed to the pigs in a liquid form. Since the pigs can consume relatively higher quality of roughages among the non-ruminants, they can be fed on good quality forages to a sizable proportion of feed. The pigs are fed normally twice a day, morning and evening. Lack of desired feed intake is indicated either poor quality of feed or ill health of the animal.

Grains like maize, oats, sorghum can make the largest part of pig feed like other non-ruminants. However, excessive feeding is unnecessary a wasteful and uneconomical. Pigs can tolerate 10-12% of crude fibre. Most concentrate feed for pigs like other non-ruminants is made of oil cakes / meals, grain by-products such as wheat bran, rice polish, dairy industry by-products such as whey and acid whey, slaughter by-products, meat meal, bone meal, fish meal and other fishing industry waste. Garbage as indicated earlier is widely used as cheap feed for pigs but has a risk of causing diseases if not properly

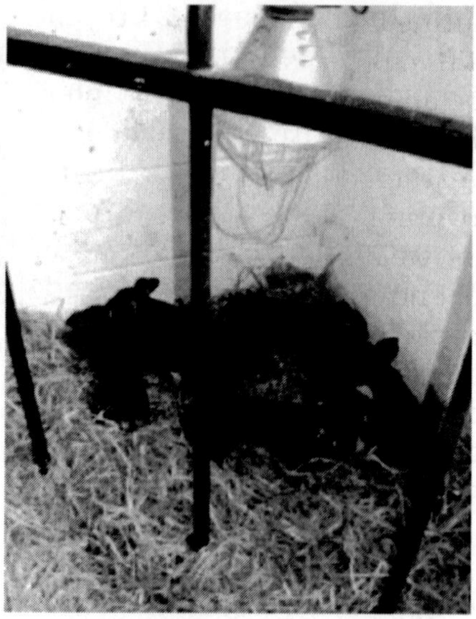

processed. In countries like North Korea, all households' kitchen waste including bones are grounded in the sink and drained in to a large collection tank from where it is transported to the pig farm. Such liquid is subjected to pressure for reducing the size of the waste feed materials and heated at a high temperature and then offered to the pigs both as feed and water source. The pig sty washings are stored in a cemented tank. The supernatant is drained and is used for culturing non-pathogenic micro-organisms and the scum is removed, heated at high temperature and used as a source of single cell protein. The rest of water with settled solid waste is fed into a fish tank to help in growth of phyto- and zoo-planktons which are source of nutrition for fish and subsequently enrich the water for irrigation of crop land etc. Thus there is an integration of household disposal with pig production, fish production and crop production which is economically and environmentally desirable.

Pre-starter feeding / creep feeding may be given to one week old piglets and should continue till weaning, which can improve their growth and survival. Such creep feed has 20-22% protein, minerals and vitamins in addition to energy and improves body weight gains and survivals of piglets. The starter/ grower ration from weaning to the age when the piglets attain 15 kg live weight and finisher ration when the piglets are of 30 kg live weight, can help in better growth, carcass yield and quality and production of lean bacon.

3.6 Transport management

In commercial pig production, the marketable piglets are transported over a long distance from the farm to regulated market for live animals to be sold for slaughter. Long distance transport is highly stressful and can lead to a loss in body weight and mortality. Regular moving and handling during the finishing period tends to reduce stress in subsequent handling and transport. The behavior of the handler is also important in maintaining the animals less disturbed during transport. Travel sickness is reflected through chewing, foaming at the mouth and sniffing at the air. To avoid stress during transport, the animal should be kept off-feed for 12-24 hours. The carrier vehicle should be thoroughly cleaned and provide protection from inclement weather. This can be done by providing bedding in the truck and covering at the top but avoiding suffocation. Sprinkling of water during hot weather, separating heavier pigs from lighter pigs and ensuring that no sharp edges of nails/ poles are present on the inner side of the truck. Suitable equipment should be available for loading and unloading. Only requisite number of pigs which can be accommodated in the space to avoid congestion should be transported. It is preferable to travel at night so that the animals reach the destination early morning and rested for some time before slaughter.

3.7 Culling

Since the herd size cannot be allowed to expand beyond the housing and management capacity; labour available and the financial resources that are easily available or can be procured, it is essential to limit the herd size. There is a definite productive age both for the breeding males and females and the optimum age of the piglets when they should be marketed for breeding/slaughter.

The sows and gilts are generally culled if they do not breed within the desired time either for the first time or after farrowing. Excessive culling can reduce the breeding herd and low culling may result in accumulation or too many low productive females. Normally sows beyond eight parities should not be retained and an ideal annual culling rate should be 40% in the herd.

The majority of females are culled due to poor fertility/fecundity, skeletal problems and old age. There are number of other reasons that may contribute excessive culling which may include sudden deaths and vulval discharge in early pregnancy. Different experts have given the culling rates ranging from 13-42 % with a average of 34 % for reproductive failure, 12% with a range from 10-24% for locomotive problems, 17.2%, ranging from 9-21% for poor litter size and 19% with a range from 10-32% for various other reasons.

Poor fertility such as due to anoestrous fourteen days after weaning in sows and 21 days in gilts will make them not fit to be retained in the herd. Similarly the females that do not become pregnant after two consecutive matings and thus found not in pig (NIPs) are culled. Males which do not show proper libido and cannot cover the requisite number of females are also culled.

Poor fecundity that is small litter size and average or higher litter mortality will also result in the culling of a breeding female.

Skeletal defects leading to lameness may be due to poor nutrition especially lack of adequate calcium, phosphorus and vitamin D. Poor availability of space, slippery floor, steep, rough or sharp structures in the pens result in poor performance. Overcrowding, frequent mixing of animals of different ages, inadequate feeding and watering space can result in poor growth and reproductive problems.

The culling rates can be reduced due to reasons other than lower values of economic characters include, chronic ill-health, permanent lameness, and consecutive small litters, structural and functional abnormalities, poor growth and survival in the piglets.

To reduce culling rates for reasons other than production efficiencies, it is necessary to improve nutrition, health and management of the herd. Regular replacement of guilts from other better performing herds especially free from any skeletal defects and better reproduction and growth can help in improving herd productivity. Sows should not normally be retained after they have produced eight litters. Generally the performance of sow in terms of reproduction and milk production is satisfactory up to six parities.

3.8 Disease management

Bacterial, viral, parasitic and nutritional factors are responsible for mortality and morbidity in pigs. Tuberculosis, swine erysipelas, pneumonia, swine dysentery are major bacterial diseases. Swine pox, FMD, swine influenza/hog cholera are common viral diseases. Internal parasitic diseases are lung-worm infection, ascariasis and tape-worms. External parasitic diseases are exanthema, mange and lice infestation. Nutritional deficiency diseases are piglet anemia, rickets, iodine deficiency, hypoglycemia and rheumatism.

These diseases can be controlled through (i) segregation, (ii) proper hygiene, (iii) providing quality feed and drinking water, (iv) proper housing, (v) continuous cleaning the floor of pig sties, (vi) rotational grazing, (vii) proper disposal of litter especially from infected animals and of carcasses, (viii) proper quarantining, (ix) regular vaccination and administration of anthelmintics against internal parasites and regular dipping/spraying with appropriate ecto-parasitic agents which will not result in toxicity to the animals and environmental pollution. In addition to the balanced feed, the fiber content should be kept low and feed should be supplemented with some green leguminous fodder. The animals may have bellowing facility in medicated water. Maintenance of proper records of reproduction and growth and their regular examination can help in determining the health status of the animals.

The vaccination schedule in pigs should be as follows:

1. After weaning (7-8 weeks) - Lapinised swine fever vaccine, 1 ml-subcutaneous provides immunity up to one year.
2. After weaning (3-6 months) vaccination against H.S. and F.M.D.
3. Normally animal should be vaccinated in March-April and six months later.

3.9 Pig mortality, causes and management

The mortality rate varies from birth to weaning (3-8weeks) to the extent of 20-30% of which neonatal averages (0-10 days - 20-30%), post weaning-grower (weaning to 2 months) and finisher (5-7/8 months or market weight 90-200 kg) 50% and total pre-natal mortality starting with parturition, and 4-5 hrs after parturition 80%. The still birth range from 4-10%. Still births may occur during the process of farrowing due to lack of adequate blood supply through placenta, or umbilical cord or cut-off of the umbilical cord due to uterine contraction during parturition leading to asphyxia. Death in sows/gilts can occur before farrowing, during farrowing and after farrowing. Post-mortem examination can indicate whether the animal was still-born or died after birth. The necropsy can indicate whether the animal was still-born from its freshness, still being contained in the membranes, may be attached to the umbilical cord, there may be discoloration of skin, muscles may be moist on incision, organs may appear fresh with large amount of yellowish secretions and the lungs are usually atelectic. If the piglet dies before birth it will show varying degree of degenerative changes including discoloration of skin and loss of fluid. In case of death in early stages of pregnancy a fully formed mummified piglet may be seen. The piglet that dies during parturition or immediately after parturition will appear fresh. The two types of dead piglets can be differentiated if the chest is opened and lungs are examined. The lungs of the true still birth pigs are dark, plum in color showing none of the pink area associated with inflation and breathing. A longer farrowing time is associated with higher rate of still birth because of disruption of the umbilical blood flow.

Still birth may result from increased age of sow, larger litter size, it has higher incidence is in purebreds and in the last third period of farrowing. The temperature of the farrowing house above 24 degree centigrade increases still birth due to difficulty of the sow to dissipate body heat and results in panting while resting during delivery. The uterine inertia often resulting from calcium deficiency results in high incidence of still births. Interruption of the blood supply to the fetus due to pressure or rupture of umbilical cord results in lack of availability of oxygen and accumulation of carbon dioxide and thus affecting the health of the fetuses. Hypothermia is a dominant cause of piglet mortality and maintenance of appropriate temperature in farrowing pen can reduce piglet mortality at birth. In case of abnormally long gestation period administration of oxytocin can help in early delivery and reduced piglet mortality. Lack of exercise of sow also results in higher incidence of still birth. Diseases like fever, mastitis, septicemia, acute stress and haemorrhage can result into excess incidence of still birth. Anaemia, Aujeszky's disease, Enteroviruses, Eperythrozoonosis, Erysipelas, Leptospirosis, Mycotoxicosis, Parvovirus, PRRS, Toxoplasmosis, Septicaemia, Swine fever and Avitaminosis result in higher incidence of still birth. The incidence of still birth can be reduced through identifying and culling of problem sows, attending cases of distocia, observing farrowing behavior, ensuring proper design of farrowing pen, monitoring farrowing and providing assistance in case of difficult farrowing. The farrowing pen should be properly heated to avoid chill but not excessive heat. Earlier records of the farrowing of the sow should be studied, haemoglobin level cheked, parasitic load reduced before parturition. Any abnormal discharge should be seen with concern and suitable corrective measures should be taken.

Gastritis, Haemorrhagic gastritis and Necrotic gastritis are caused by Streptococcus species and amount to 5.80 and 1.02% mortality respectively. Further enteritis is caused by *E. coli* which causes 5.11% mortality, Diphtheritic enteritis is caused by Salmonella and results in 12.62% mortality. Haemorrahagic enteritis, Necrotic enteritis, Gastroenteritis are caused by *Salmonella* and *E. coli* spp. results in 0.68, 0.68 and 5.11% mortality. Pathogenic condition/diseases such as Pneumonia, Bronchopneumonia, Fibrinopurulent pneumonia are caused by *Streptococcus and Staphylococcus spp.* and *E. coli* spp. causing

2.04% mortality. Haemorrhagic pneumonia caused by *Pasteurella, Streptococcus* and *Staphylococcus spp.* results in 4.43% mortality. Suppurative pneumonia caused by *Streptococcus* and *Staphylococcus spp.* accounts for 3.4%, Swine fever associated with *E. coli* and Salmonella for 36.53%, Septicaemia caused by *E. coli* and *Streptococcus species* for 1.70, meningitis caused by *Streptococcus species* for 0.34 %, mycotoxicity caused by Aflatoxin for 0.68%. Non-infectious causes such as traumatic injury, stampede or crushing by overlying, congenital anomalies and Inanition result in 2.38, 0.34 and 8.19% mortality, NAD and Autolysis resulting in 3.07 and 1.70 indicating total of 13.62% mortality on the basis of 293 piglets born.

3.10 Pre-weaning mortality

Next to the pre and antenatal mortality, pre-weaning mortality from birth to weaning is also high with almost two piglets per litter lost during this period. Therefore, efforts are required not only to reduce ante and post-natal mortality but also pre-weaning mortality. The weaning weigh is not only responsible for post-weaning mortality but is important in determining post weaning growth and carcass yield and quality.

3.11 Factors affecting pre-weaning mortality

i) Feed intake during gestation especially later part which determines the birth weight of piglets and milk yield of the dam and thus the young survival and growth.

ii) Farrowing crate design is closely related to neo-natal mortality due to trauma, compared to sows farrowing in un-confined conditions.

iii) Spatial arrangements. Two spatial arrangements can be identified in farrowing pens, a safe zone for the piglets to rest and interaction zone where they interact with the mother during suckling and run a risk of being crushed under the dams weight when it changes its posture or sits down disregarding the presence of the piglets.

iv) Maintaining appropriate temperature in the farrowing pen which should be 30-34 degree centigrade. When the ambient temperature is below 34 °C, the young piglets are subjected to cold stress.

v) Fostering effective care by dam has a marked effect on the pre-weaning mortality and growth. The major factors governing the mortality are the extent of variations in weight and size of the piglets. Majority of low weigh piglets cannot compete for the dam's teats and thus can not suckle sufficient milk. Such piglets should be artificially fed and provided proper protection from inclement weather.

vi) Good shed hygiene is important in reducing infections in pre-weaning pigs and thus lowering mortality. Proper cleaning and disinfection of sheds is necessary to reduce microbial infection and pre-weaning mortality.

vii) Litter size increases with age and with parity and this further increases the piglet losses due to competition for the mother's milk and attention. Small and weaker pigs can not compete for reaching the udder and thus starve to death.

viii) About 15% piglets die due to overlying of the sow on them.

Farrowing house management is crucial for young survival and should involve assuring clean and cool drinking water availability especially during hot summer days. Feed intake should also be assessed and generally a target of 6-7 kg per lactating sow between farrowing and weaning should be assured. Fecal consistency and color and consistency of urine should be observed, vomition, skin injuries, bloat /tympanists and lameness should be observed and necessary ameliorative measures taken. Rectal temperature should not exceed 4 °C above normal even in hot weather. The respiration rate during resting should range between 12-30 per minute. Post farrowing stress should be minimized through proper management to reduce incidence of infectious and non-infectious diseases.

Non-infectious causes of mortality of piglets relate to i) crushing or traumatic injury, ii) naval bleeding, iii) anaemia, iv) hypoglycemia because of starvation, v) congenital abnormalities such as eye- defects, cystic kidneys, vi) splay leg and vii) savaged by dam. Infectious diseases are TGE, diarrhoea caused by *Rota virus/E. coli/Salmonella/ Streptococcus spp.*, pneumonia caused by *Streptococcus, Staphylococcus* and *Pasteurella* species and mycotic infection resulting in gastritis.

The new born piglets require i) good physical environment and should be maintained under thermo-neutral conditions and further prevented from draught. ii) They should be provided with adequate feed and water in addition to suckling of the dam and high energy and protein density creep feed from two weeks after birth. iii) They should be protected from infectious and non-infectious diseases and mechanical injuries. To avoid their moving off from the dam, guard railing should be provided.

3.12 Neo-natal mortality

Non-infectious causes result in 22.8% mortality of which the major component (17%) is due to overlaying of dams, 4% due to biting injury, 2% by savaging by dam. This is followed by hypo-glycaemia (17%), congenital abnormalities (14%) with 7% eye defect, 6% cystic kidneys and atresia, inanition (5.5%). Infectious diseases include bacterial diseases resulting in 18% mortality of which *E.coli* (9.9%), *Streptococci* (8%), mycotic infections (4.35%) of which *Mucormycotic gastritis* is (4%), rhizopus and *Candida gastritis* (0.99%) and multiple causes (6.4%). Pneumo-enteritis due to *Streptocococcus* and *E.coli* result in 2.5% mortality. Eye defects and hypoglycemia results in 2%, Streptococcal pneumonia, hernia and hypoglycemia 1.98%, hypoglycemia and cystic kidneys 0.99% and unclassified diseases 10.89%.

Birth weight is an important factor in determining mortality, it ranges from 6.5% in bodyweight group (1.61-1.80kg to 56% in weight group of 0.90kg and less). The mortality is also higher in heavier birth weight piglets.

Physiological characters of the neonates related to young mortality are:

i) **Fat content:** The neonate has low fat deposit (1% of live weight) and therefore it mostly relies on the dam's milk for its survival.

ii) **Carbohydrate contents:** The level of liver glycogen at birth is only sufficient for meeting the energy requirements for 15-24 hours after birth. Since gluconeogenesis mechanism is not developed in the liver up to seven days of age, death is inevitable if constant supply of easily utilizable carbohydrates through dam's milk to the young piglets in not made.

iii) Ability to regulate body temperature in neonate piglets is highly limited which makes them very susceptible to energy deficiency due to incapability of regulating temperature and thus enabling proper suckling.

iv) The milk of sow has low iron content and this condition results in piglet anemia unless supplementary iron is provided.

v) Deprivation of colostrums to weak and debilitated piglets due to lack of competition with healthier and heavier piglets results in starvation deaths.

Biological behavior in terms of (i) litter size which normally ranges between 8-10 in indigenous pigs and any larger litter will result in greater competition for milk and higher mortality in weaker piglets, (ii) the birth weight of piglets is determined by the age of the dam, its body weight at farrowing, ante and post natal feed intake and body condition. Thus piglets in large litters born to younger and poor conditioned dams will have higher mortality and (iii) The age of the young affects the mortality which is highest on the first day after birth (13%) which includes still births. The losses decline from second day onward and are 3% on 2nd and 3rd day and 2% on 4th day followed by a further decline up to 0.02% from 28-154 days of age. The low birth weight, larger competition among littermates in larger litters for milk and higher susceptibility to infectious and non-infectious diseases result in higher mortality and morbidity. Larger number of deaths take place between removal of the foetal membranes of the young and the first feed. There may be partial expansion of lungs resulting in respiratory distress which is more common in low birth weight piglets especially born in larger litters and to younger and lighter sows which have not been fed and looked after well in pre-partum period. Further infection due to *E.coli* and *Clostridium perfringens* (Type C) occurs within 36-48 hours and results in heavy mortality. TGE, vomiting and wasting diseases, *Streptococcal septicaemia* and *Actinobacillus* due to a *A. suis* can cause serious neo-natal mortality.

Clinical symptoms

Weak piglets which have survived immediately after birth may be unable to compete with other litter mates for suckling. This may be due to partial expansion of the lungs resulting from to high rate of shallow respiration. Similarly those with weak legs are less vigorous and thus have difficulty in reaching the mother and thus competing for milk with normal and heavier piglets. The clinical signs of hypoglycaemia develop and ultimately result in death. Under weight piglets because of higher competition with normal piglets aimlessly wander for feed. Normal piglets may also develop hypoglycaemia if agalactia is present in the dams. Agalactia and mastitis may result after feeding of colostrums and may results in neonatal mortality. Infections like *E.coli, C. perfringens* type C are usually present. Crushing by the mother is also an important cause of death in weaker piglets.

The occurrence of abnormal neonatal mortality can be easily identified by presence of a number of dead piglets and if they are not readily removed can be scavenged by predators or removed by workers to avoid being blamed for negligence. The neonatal and prenatal deaths should be distinguished when the piglets have escaped the membranes; tips of the toes wear away and leave the hooves unprotected. If the tips are still present and the piglet have not walked should be classified as having died during intra-partum period. When the farrowing is closely watched, the clinical signs leading to mortality can indicate the cause which may be preventable.

Treatment of remaining piglets of the affected litters should be carried out through ensuring warmth and helping the weaker piglets in consuming colostrums. If they cannot suckle, they may be artificially fed colostrums and fostered on another recently farrowed lactating sow. The piglets which are too light in weight and extremely weak with little chance of survival should be humanely killed. Similarly the piglets with congenital defects or incurable injury occurring during parturition or post-partum period should be destroyed. Proper care during the farrowing and ensuring proper suckling of all the piglets can help in reducing piglet mortality. Prevention of mastitis in sows through proper treatment and preventive maternal vaccination against early infection in piglets can help in reducing their mortality.

Crushing and traumatic injury on the first day of life result in major piglets' mortality. Heavier and slightly sick dam are more likely to cause death in piglets, especially if the floor is uncomfortable and pig sty in not sufficiently warm and guard railing are not provided along the walls for piglets to move after suckling.

Navel bleeding should be stopped and the navel cord disinfected. The litter size may be equalized among sows farrowing within 24 hours. Heavier piglets can be more easily fostered. Piglet anemia is a major cause of piglet mortality and morbidity as the milk produced by the sow is deficient in iron. Iron-dextran injection intramuscular can help in providing necessary iron to the piglets. 150-200 mg of iron dextran for 2-3 days after birth can prevent piglet anemia. Iron can also be given through feed and drinking water. Hypoglycemia in newborn piglets results due to poor availability of stored glycogen. Further the fat content in piglets is less than 1% of the weight and cannot be mobilized to meet the energy requirements especially if the piglets do not receive adequate milk from their dam or are exposed to cold. They have poor body energy reserves and the blood glucose level fall dramatically after birth. The lowering of blood glucose results in lethargy and lack of efforts to suckle which result in ultimate death unless it is corrected by nursing or oral or intravenous administration of glucose.

During suckling period, piglet scours result in major mortality and morbidity. It is caused by *E.coli* which are naturally present in GI tract of all mammals. Watery yellowish faeces from 1-4 days of age and then subsequently at 3 weeks of age and at weaning are often observed in poorly managed herds. The early suckling of piglets and protection from infection and inclement weather can help in reducing piglet mortality and morbidity. A dry warm draught free environment for rearing piglets is important in reducing diarrhea, TGE and swine dysentery.

Clip needle teeth, notch ear for identification and dock the tail in first few days. Creep feeding should be started as early as possible to improve live weight gains and reduce mortality and morbidity specially in weaner pigs. In addition to the creep feed some green fodder should be offered to piglets before weaning.

Piglets can be weaned early if they are well managed and have been provided with creep feed with high energy and protein and some green fodder. Attention should also be given to availability to clean drinking water. It is extremely important to have a dry warm/ well insulated but well ventilated house. For weaned piglets which should be housed in groups of 20-25 in a run. The animals should be grouped by size and animals of similar size/ weight should be housed together. A space of 3-4 ft^2 should be allowed per weaner. Weaners suffer from high parasitic load immediately after weaning. Examination of EPG and administration of specific / broad spectrum anthelmintic can help in reducing gastrointestinal parasitism. Mange and other ectoparasite can also result in serious morbidity and the piglets should be properly sprayed with appropriate and preferably broad spectrum anti-ectoparasitic agent.

3.13 Management of weaner pigs

Weaning is a stressful experience for young piglets because of the loss of the care of the mother and of the suckling which in addition to providing milk, promotes close physical and psychological relationship with the mother. However, if the weaning is done early and the piglets from 15 days after birth are provided creep feed, the adverse effect of weaning can be minimized. This will reduce mortality and morbidity in weaned piglets and thus post- weaning economic losses and improve post- weaning survival and growth.

Conventionally the weaning is done at 3-5 weeks of age but it can be done as early as 10 days to 3 weeks. Specialized weaning segregated early weaning (SEW) and modified early weaning (MEW) are recommended. Conventionally, the weaning is done when the piglets have reached a weight of 5-10 kg. Weaning is an integral part of the management and would depend on the breed, litter size and weight of the piglets attained. If desired weight has been attained early and the piglets have been accustomed to creep feed and separation from dam at least for sometimes the effect of the weaning will not be adverse on growth and survival of the piglets. The lactation yield starts declining after 5 weeks and early weaning and proper post-weaning management will not only improve survival and live weight gains and allow earlier marketing of saleable piglets or breeding of selected gilts. This will help in having an additional farrowing in a year and thus additional piglets from the same sow in a year. This may also ultimately help in increasing selection intensity and genetic gains in economic characters related to meat production through selection and if desired through mating lines selected for different economic traits especially those which are negatively related.

Normally, piglets reach 4-5 kg live weight at 2-3 weeks of age when their digestive system can handle more complex carbohydrates and they can develop heat regulating capabilities. Thus they are capable to better adjust to post weaning environment even if the weaning is done early. However the weaning prior to 3-4 weeks is not common as the piglets have not developed proper immunological and physiological maturity and can thus not able to stand extreme physical environmental conditions. The use of specialized weaning facilities can help considerably in early weaning, these may involve starting of early creep feeding, proper protection against prevalent infectious diseases and parasites and inclement weather. They should increase the number of farrowing per unit time and thus produce more piglets for marketing per unit time.

3.14 Specialized weaning

Segregated early weaning (SEW) can be practiced at a suitable early age usually less than 18 days and removing the piglets from the breeding herd immediately after weaning for eliminating or at least reducing the disease incidence in weaner piglets.

3.15 Medicated early weaning (MEW)

To obtain pathogen free pigs specially from endemic diseases the sows are administered large doses of antibiotics when they enter the farrowing pens until their piglets are weaned which is done at 5 days of age and the piglets are moved to an isolated early weaning unit and are administered from birth up to 10 days of age with similar drugs as given to the sows to keep them free from disease.

There are however problems associated with early weaning which causes stressful conditions for piglets and may result in bad habits such as cannibalism, depressed growth and scouring. A critical factor in early weaning and supplementing with creep feeding during suckling is the limitation of the creep feed consumed. Early creep feeding accelerates development of digestive system and thus help in improved feed intake and growth. The use of high energy sources such as molasses and jaggery can be advantageous to meet high energy requirements.

After weaning there is a change in social behavior and development of dominance/ peck order within the litter and the piglets with lower body weight are put to a disadvantage in feeding and have higher susceptibility to environmental and disease hazards. If the piglets are separated by size and sex and moved to a new strange surroundings where they spend the next few days establishing a new social (peck) order and adjust to a new environment. This adjustment may lead to reduced feed intake and thus impose nutritional stress and also may impede their growth and development.

At weaning the piglets are to adjust largely from liquid to solid feed unless they have already fed creep feed. The development of gastro-intestinal system to the new feed takes a few days when the nutrient availability may be lesser than required and may result in loss of body weight. This may also result in poor disease resistance due to antigenic reaction of feed.

The digestive system of piglets is geared to handle milk and milk based diet. The pigs weaned at 28 days or more have higher capability to handle non-milk carbohydrates and protein than pigs weaned at 14 days of age.

The neonates have no protective immunity at birth and rely on the consumption of colostrum for the transfer of passive immunity from the mother. This immunity lasts for 10 to 14 days after birth. But the piglets do not attain capability of their own immune system before 21-28 days of age. Therefore piglets weaned early (14-28 days of age) are at a risk because of lack of their own immune capability. There are however effective vaccines available against most common diseases and can be administered both to pre-weaning and post-weaning piglets.

When fed only twice a day, piglets tends to use large quantities of feed in a short period of time and thus void a large quantity undigested feed in fecal matter. This also results in heavy loading of the digestive and absorption ability of the gastro-intestinal tract. Feed may pass too quickly through the GI tract and thus may be available to micro-organism in the lower part of gut. However, when the same feed is offered in small quantities and a number of times and at regular intervals, the GI tract empties intermittently and is gentler to the GI tract and the enzymes to act for a longer period and ensure proper digestion of feed.

The stomach pH in pigs varies along the GI tract, it is more acidic in stomach due to the presence of hydrochloric acid which helps in protein digestion and also helps in preventing growth of pathogenic bacteria. When the pig is fed, the pH changes towards the pH of the feed, the stomach secretes HCl and pH again falls. If the feed is eaten in large quantities and at frequent intervals, the stomach pH tends to remain higher for a longer period. This allows bacteria to multiply and travel to the intestine and along with the undigested feed cause the growth of *E. coli* which results in scours and even death.

The pre–weaning management would involve offering fresh pig starter feed daily from as early as to 4-5 days. This will reduce the effect of the diet change at weaning and promote maturity of gastric enzyme system. If the weaning is done around 24 – 28 days an intake of 600 g of creep feed should be ensured before weaning. Adequate water should also be offered. All marking operation for identification, castration, docking should be carried out prior to weaning. Antibiotics should be supplemented in the feed of weaners both before and after weaning. Feed should not be changed frequently. While mixing litters at weaning allow them to run together before weaning.

At weaning the piglets should be taken away from their dam so that they cannot see or smell the mother. While separating from the mother, mother should be removed first and then the individual piglets are handled preferably individually without causing serious stress. A long bamboo with a crook may be used to catch the piglets or they may be driven into a blind alley in the creep area to help in trapping them. The piglets should be held under the chest with both the hands and placed into the barrow or trolley which may contain wood shavings or rice husks. The trolley should be covered with a lid to avoid the piglets jumping out.

Early weaning helps in early breeding of sows and thus producing more litters per year. The early weaning can result in a depression in sows productivity and failing to return to oestrus after weaning if not handled properly.

The smaller the piglets, higher is the risks if feed is not adequate and physical environment is not comfortable. Specialized pens or even crouches are very useful in handling weaner pigs. Smaller piglets have lower feed intake and require higher temperature at weaning.

Weaner pens should be clean, dry, drought free and avoid large temperature fluctuations. Deep litter of straw may be provided to keep the piglets warm and comfortable. Weaner houses may have all in and all out arrangements. In deep litter system, provision of slow upped insulated hovers with well straw bedded areas provide comfortable conditions. It will be desirable if extra feeding and watering trays are provided close to the entrance in the first weak post weaning.

While ensuring appropriate temperature, ventilation and hygiene, space should be provided according to the weight / size of the animal, which may range from 0.09 square meter for a pig weighing 5 kg to 0.37 m^2 for a pig weighing 35 kg. In deep litter system, the space provided may be 1.5 times larger. Normally less than 20 piglets per group are maintained in conventional housing system, but can go up from 125-250 under a deep litter system. The larger the size of the group, greater will be the competition for space both in the pen and for water and feed. This will adversely affect the growth and survival of weaker piglets.

3.16 Feeding weaners

While weaning at 3-4 weeks of age the piglets should have attained 300-350 g average daily gain (ADG). After weaning there is a sudden reduction in ADG which may go down to 100 g. A quick recovery will depend on the quality of feed, physical environment and space and skill of the handler. The first few hours after weaning are crucial and weaners should be provided with comfort in the new shelter and given proper feed and water. The stress leads to *E. coli* infection, resulting in diarrhea and destabilizing the intestinal flora. It may take 10-14 days for the animal to come out of the post-weaning depression.

Continuation of the same high quality creep feeding 10-14 days after weaning and gradual change in the feed composition and an increase in feed offered can help. The feed offered should be increased from 150 g per day in the first week to 250- 300 g per day in the second week. In the first week, feed may be offered in flat trays.

3.17 Water supply

Ensure clean fresh water to piglets all the time. Water should be free from bacterial contamination and should be soft. On an average two litre per day for a piglet up to 20 kg live weight is sufficient provided in the drinker for four to five piglets. Addition of electrolytes can be helpful during early life. Medication can also be done through drinking water. The drinker should be covered except for the openings for the piglets to drink to avoid spoilage of water. Water temperature should preferably between 16-18 °C during winter.

3.18 Health and hygiene

Weaners are highly susceptible to most infectious systemic diseases immediately after weaning and high level of hygiene and protection against infectious diseases and internal and external parasites is required. Poor performing piglets should preferably be culled. Sick animals should be isolated and treated and mixed with the other weaners when they are healthy. Animals should be regularly examined for their health and growth.

Since the young piglets specially the females will provide replacement for breeding females, greater care in their management, particularly housing, feeding and health care should be taken so as to reduce morbidity and mortality and ensure proper growth and attainment of early puberty. The economic returns from a pig farm as well as genetic progress through selection largely depends on reproductive efficiency of sow and must be maximized through proper housing/feeding and health care. Proper protection from inclement weather through appropriate housing, maintenance of hygiene through proper cleaning and disinfection and ensuring proper nutrition.

❑❑❑

CHAPTER-4

Pig Nutrition
(Nutritional Requirements of Pigs under Intensive and Extensive Production Systems and Ration Formulation)

Pig production is an important enterprise for rural employment and incomes and providing protein rich food utilizing various plants and animal wastes because it can breed two to three times in a year depending upon the age at weaning of the litter. Pig production so far has been an occupation mostly part time of economically and socially poor people utilizing plant and animal wastes either directly through scavenging by the pigs which would require with roaming around large areas in rural and peri-urban populations or fed on food waste collected from different sources e.g. eateries (hotels and restaurants), vegetable and fruit markets and cereal, vegetable and fruits and meat processing factories. Pig is an efficient utilizer of feed and has a higher feed conversion ratio except chicken.

Efficient utilization of feed nutrients depends on adequate supply of energy, protein with essential amino acids, which is of paramount importance in determining the efficiency of pig production. Nutrient requirement depends on body size, growth rate and genetic potential for growth, efficiency of feed conversion, carcass yield and meat quality. The physical environment viz relative humidity, solar radiation, wind velocity and rainfall affect the production especially when the pigs are not adequately housed to protect them from inclement weather. Considering the environmental conditions, the nutrient supply can be regulated. Feeding standards cannot be applied to all agro-ecological and production systems. Scientific knowledge on nutrient supply is essential to maximize nutrient utilization and minimize their excretion. It is therefore necessary to understand the nutrient requirements of different breeds or breed crosses, as the litter which can be increased through selection and following proper mating system for exploiting both additive and non-additive (heterosis resulting from dominance and epistatic effects of genes and due to linkage of different genes affecting the economic characters. It will therefore require that in recommending the nutrient/feeding standards and the feed resources that should be utilized, the genetic background of the pigs involved, physical environment, management system, feed resources available and their nutrient value and the market demand for the live weight and quality of pork which will differ due to subsequent processing and marketing, should be considered.

4.1 Feeding systems

Pigs in rural and peri-urban areas are mostly reared under scavenging conditions. More recently due to efforts in genetic improvement through provision of boars of improved indigenous or exotic breeds or their crosses for breeding, with indigenous non-descript pigs and advise the pig keepers to feed them on house hold wastes and wastes from vegetable and fruit market, small and large eateries (hotel) and other meat, vegetable and fruit processing industries. However, under intensive production system primarily involving purebred exotics or their crosses with indigenous or among exotic breeds and provide proper shelters and balanced compounded feed. The latter is primarily based on cereal and oil seed processing by-products, some coarse cereals, root crops like sweet potato.

4.2 Creep feed

Practice of early weaning of piglets at six weeks of age and even earlier is becoming a common practice in western commercial pig production systems and is also being introduced under Indian conditions for more efficient live weight gains and carcass yield and quality and thus providing optimum and earlier economic returns. Generally, the piglets are weaned at eight weeks of age under intensive feeding and management system. However, weaning is advantageous on weight basis rather than on age basis as traditionally practiced. The earlier gains are more efficient and the feed is primarily utilized for development of muscles rather than fat. Split weaning in larger litters is often practiced where the heavier piglets are weaned early and put under intensive feeding and the weaker piglets are allowed to suckle their dams and are also allowed on creep feed (pre-starter feed) till they reach desired live weight and are subsequently put on intensive feeding. Creep is essential for suckling piglets for faster growth and attainment of satisfactory weaning weight. Piglets should have easy access to creep feed for *ad-lib* intake. Creep feed should contain 20% DCP and 3265 kcal ME per kg. The feed should be fortified with minerals and vitamins. Creep feed generally has added ferrous sulphate in the ratio of 9:1 to prevent piglet anemia. Creep feed is introduced from 7-14 days of age and is continued to be fed till weaning. Piglets fed on creep feed attain live weight of 12-15 kg at 8 weeks of age in exotic breeds like Landrace and Yorkshire. During suckling period piglets are more prone to anemia. A dose of iron injected (iron dextran) at 4th and 14th day will help in prevent in piglet anemia. An alternate method of supply of iron to the new born piglet is to paint the sow's udder with liquid oral iron supplement.

4.3 Feeding growing piglets

After weaning of piglets which are supplemented with creep feed when they attain 12-15 kg live weight at 8 weeks of age are switched over to grower ration. They consume considerably more feed. With careful feeding management, piglets can attain on an average 20 kg live weight and would look thrifty in appearance as they have almost passed the nutritionally critical period and will perform relatively better on even a simpler ration under optimum management.

4.4 Feeding finisher piglets

On attainment of average body weight of 30-50 kg, the piglets are switched over to finisher ration till they attain market weight of 60-70 kg. Marketing based on this slaughter weight is more economical than at a higher market weight (90 kg) normally recommended in western countries. For the indigenous pig, a slaughter weight of 45-50 kg is generally recommended. The finisher piglets should be fed on lower energy diet and that too on strictly pre-determined basis to make meat production more economical.

4.5 Feeding of pregnant and lactating sows

Finisher pigs are selected for breeding as sows / boars and are continued to be fed on high level of nutrition also with high level of vitamins. Feeding of pregnant sows and gilts should match with their nutrient requirement. The feed offered should be restricted to 2-2.5 kg per day because higher quantity of feed may lead to increased embryonic mortality. The recommended ration is 2.0 kg of grower/ finisher ration containing 16% CP, 3000 kcal DE / kg feed with 0.7% lysine for 15 days till finishing. On the day of farrowing 250 g of wheat bran should be given for ensuring proper initiation of lactation. Thereafter for the next 3 days increasing quantity of above recommended ration should be offered in a manner that the sow could consume at least 2 kg feed. From 5th day onwards after freshening, the sow should be fed to appetite (*ad. lib.*). The lactating sow should be fed for the early recovery of body weight lost at farrowing. 3.5 kg feed with 0.2 kg per suckling piglet should be provided.

4.6 Feeding of boars

Boars used for breeding should be fed on a finisher ration, but the quantity should be restricted to 2.5 kg/head/day. In addition green fodder such as berseem /lucerne may be given to the boars. 1.5-1.8 kg of grower/finisher ration with 16% CP, 3000 kcal DE/kg diet with additional 0.7% lysine given to the boars when not being used for service.

4.7 Feeding of grower pigs

Growing pigs of exotic breeds are fed according to their requirement in different growth phases which depends on age and live weight. Four different phases viz. 15-20, 20-35, 35-60 and 60-100 kg up to 100 kg are generally recommended. Others recommend six growing phases viz. 3-5, 5-10, 10-20, 20-50, 50-80 and 80-120 kg. Under Indian conditions, three stages viz. weaning (5-12 kg), growing (12-50 kg) and finishing (50-100 kg) up to live weight of 100 kg are recommended. Phasing of feeding varies with live weight, mainly due to differences arising from genetic back ground (breed and breed cross), climatic conditions and desired target live weight. The requirement of CP, TDN and DE along with essential amino acids for maintenance and growth are DE 123.3 kcal (516 kJ) to 167.8 kcal (702 kJ) per kg metabolic body weight. The estimates from the whole database on feeding trials is 164.4 kcal (688 kJ/ kg metabolic body weight). These values are higher than recommended by Agricultural Research Council (ARC) and Nutritional Research Council (NRC).

Since the nutritional requirements as mentioned earlier would vary widely according to genotype, management conditions, environmental conditions and desired final live weight, the recommendation should be considered as guide and should be changed according to the new feed resources available, the genetic constitution of the pigs to be raised and the market demand for live weight at marketing and carcass yield and quality.

4.8 Nutrient requirement for exotic purebred, crossbred and indigenous breeds

The exotic breeds of pigs introduced in the country are Landrace and White Yorkshire. They are essentially maintained at Institutional breeding farms for research for producing breeding boars both purebreds and crossbred with indigenous breeds. The exotic pigs attain an average body weight of 74 kg at 32 weeks of age. Dietary requirements on *ad. lib.* feeding of exotic breeds under Indian conditions are given in Table 2.

Table 2. Dietary requirements (as fed basis) of exotic pigs under Indian agro-climatic conditions

Age (weeks)	**8 to 16**	**17 to 24**	**25 to 32**
Body weight (kg)	10 to 25	26 to 48	49 to 75
Av weight (kg)	17.7	36.3	61.0
BW gain (g/d)	255	410	475
Av daily feed intake (g/d)	960	1,560	2,170
Feed: Gain	3.79	3.80	4.58
Nutrient requirements			
DE (kcal / kg diet)	3,000	3,180	2,600
DE (kJ / kg diet)	12,579	13,311	10,883
ME (kcal / kg diet)	2,886	3,054	2,497
ME (kJ / Kg diet)	12,075	12,779	10,447
CP (%)	18.4	16.7	15.0
Lysine (%)	0.70	0.65	0.60
Methionine (%)	0.56	0.51	0.50
Methionine + Cysteine (%)	0.29	0.29	0.26
Cysteine (%)	0.85	0.80	0.76
Threonine (%)	0.62	0.62	0.62
Tryptophan (%)	0.19	0.19	0.19

(*Source:* Nutrient Requirements of Pig, Indian Council of Agricultural Research, New Delhi, 2013.

In case of indigenous breeds based on the observations made at AICRP on pigs and with ADG of 0.152, 0.186 and 0.262 kg during 6-20, 20-30 and 30-60 weeks of age. The nutrient requirement were calculated for three phases of growth and are given in Table 3 and 4.

Table 3. Body weight changes (kg) of indigenous pigs

Age (week)	Jabalpur	Tirupati	Izatnagar	Khanapara	Average
Birth	0.7	0.78	0.68	0.83	0.75
4	3.61	4.07	3.95	3.96	3.90
8	7.59	8.12	7.32	8.01	7.76
12	9.3	11.47	10.75	10.98	10.63
16	13.16	15.83	14.7	17.39	15.27
20	16.27	22.47	20.81	22.59	20.54
24	21.99	30.82	25.5	28.36	26.67
28	24.72	35.24	31.35	32.56	30.97

(*Source:* Nutrient Requirements of Pig, Indian Council of Agricultural Research, New Delhi, 2013)

Table 4. Dietary requirements (as fed-basis) of desi (native) pigs

Age (weeks)	8 to 20			21 to 28		29 to 32	
Body weight (kg)	6 to 20			21 to 30		31 to 40	
Daily feed intake (g/d)	610	650	700	900	950	1,350	1,400
Feed: Gain	4.01	4.30	4.57	4.86	5.10	5.18	5.33
Nutrient requirements							
DE (kcal/kg diet)	3,170	2,950	2,780	3,185	3,030	2,570	2,495
DE (kJ/kg diet)	13,252	12,350	11,622	13,325	12,698	10,741	10,439
ME (kcal/kg diet)	3,040	2,830	2,670	3,060	2,900	2,470	2,395
ME (kJ/kg diet)	12,720	11,857	11,160	12,792	12,190	10,311	10,022
CP (%)	20	18.65	17.50	18.70	17.80	15.30	14.95
Lysine (%)	0.83	0.77	0.73	0.99	0.94	0.79	0.76
Methionine (%)	0.61	0.57	0.54	0.61	0.58	0.59	0.57
Methionine + Cysteine (%)	0.92	0.86	0.81	0.94	0.89	0.84	0.81
Cysteine (%)	0.65	0.60	0.57	0.69	0.65	0.68	0.66
Threonine (%)	0.31	0.60	0.57	0.34	0.65	0.24	0.66
Tryptophan (%)	0.20	0.19	0.18	0.20	0.19	0.25	0.24

(*Source:* Nutrient Requirements of Pig, Indian Council of Agricultural Research, New Delhi, 2013)

Exotic x Indigenous (mostly non-descript) crossbred pigs are most widely used for commercial pork production. Under different feeding condition, live weight gain varies from 43-60 kg at 32 weeks of age. Landrace crosses however could attain 110 kg live weight at 32 weeks. The crossbred pigs attain higher body weight even than the exotic breed in intensive management under Indian agro-climatic conditions. The recommendations of NRC have generally been used the recommended nutrient requirements for maintenance and ADG in three phases i.e. 8-16, 16-24 and 24-32 weeks of age. The nutritive requirements for the crossbred are presented in Table 5.

Table 5. Dietary nutrient requirements (as fed-basis) of crossbred (Landrace x desi) pregnant gilts

Days of Gestation	0 to 75	75 to 111/114
Body weight (kg)	78.00 to 112.3	120.5 to 130.6
Average Weight (kg)	94.3	126.3
Average Daily Feed Intake (kg)	2.20	2.50
Feed: Gain	4.80	5.20
DE kcal/kg	3,440	3,420
DE MJ/Kg	14.40	14.30
ME kcal/kg	3,300	3,280
ME MJ/kg	13.84	13.74
CP (%)	18.84	18.92
Lysine (%)	0.80	0.83
Methionine (%)	0.65	0.70
Methionine + Cysteine (%)	0.99	0.99
Cysteine (%)	0.34	0.35
Threonine (%)	0.70	0.72
Tryptophan (%)	0.21	0.22

(*Source:* Nutrient Requirements of Pig, Indian Council of Agricultural Research, New Delhi, 2013)

Crossbred (Landrace x Indigenous) lactating sows

The nutrient requirements have been worked out in two phases i.e. up to 21 days and last 35 days before weaning. Nutrient requirements (g/day) of sows were calculated separately for maintenance and average daily loss in body weight. The DE, CP and limiting amino acids as recommended by NRC i.e. maintenance of metabolic body weight and growth are presented in Table 6.

Table 6. Dietary nutrient requirements (as fed-basis) of cross-bred lactating sow

	Days of lactation					
	0 to 21			**21 to 56**		
Body weight (kg)	120 to 112 (Mean 115.6)			112 to 99 (Mean 105.9)		
Average daily feed intake (kg/d)	3.80	4.30	4.800	3.80	4.30	4.80
DE (kcal/kg diet)	3,400	3,000	2,700	3,400	3,000	2,700
DE (MJ/kg diet)	14.20	12.50	11.30	14.20	12.50	11.30
ME (kcal/kg diet)	3,264	2,880	2,592	3,264	2,880	2,592
ME (MJ/kg diet)	13.70	12.05	10.80	13.70	12.05	10.80
CP (%)	21.80	19.20	17.30	21.10	18.60	16.80
Lysine (%)	1.10	0.97	0.87	1.04	0.92	0.82
Methionine (%)	0.57	0.50	0.45	0.53	0.48	0.43
Methionine + Cysteine (%)	0.78	0.69	0.62	0.78	0.69	0.62
Threonine (%)	0.74	0.65	0.59	0.71	0.63	0.57
Tryptophan (%)	0.23	0.20	0.18	0.22	0.19	0.17

(*Source:* Nutrient Requirements of Pig, Indian Council of Agricultural Research, New Delhi, 2013)

The growth potentiality of crossbred pigs (Landrace x native and Large White Yorkshire x native) reared under different crossbreeding programmes varied, ranging from a live weight of 43 kg (lower to medium growth potential) to 56 kg (medium to higher growth potential) at 32 weeks of age. However, the Landrace crossbred pigs maintained at IVRI attained an average live weight of 110 kg at 32 weeks of age, as it contained more than 75% of exotic inheritance. Requirements of crossbred pigs having lower to medium growth potential are presented in Table 6, medium to higher growth potential in Table 7 and higher growth potential in Table 8.

Table 7. Dietary requirements (as fed basis) of crossbred pigs having lower to medium growth potential

Age (weeks)	8 to 20	21 to 24	25 to 32
Body weight (kg)	9 to 22	23 to 28	29 to 43
Av weight (kg)	15.64	25	36
BW gain (g/d)	155	224	263
Av daily feed intake (g/d)	610	1120	1430
Feed: Gain	3.98	5.0	5.0

Nutrient requirement			
DE (Kcal/kg diet)	3,345	2,727	2,377
DE (KJ/Kg diet)	13,993	11,408	9,944
ME (Kcal/kg diet)	3,210	2,617	2,282
ME (KJ/Kg diet)	13,433	10,951	9,546
CP (%)	21.4	15.2	14.1
Lysine (%)	0.91	0.77	0.81
Methionine (%)	0.65	0.48	0.53
Methionine + Cysteine (%)	0.98	0.76	0.77
Cysteine (%)	0.33	0.27	0.23
Threonine (%)	0.68	0.57	0.62
Tryptophan (%)	0.22	0.17	0.23

Source: Paul *et al.* (2007), NRC (1998), ARC (1981)

Table 8. Dietary requirements (as fed basis) of crossbred pigs having medium to higher growth potential

Age (weeks)	8 to 16	17 to 24	25 to 32
Body weight (kg)	10 to 21	22 to 38	39 to 56
Av weight (kg)	15.52	29.15	46.56
BW gain (g/d)	189	298	323
Av daily feed intake (g/d)	640	1,350	1,760
Feed: Gain	3.37	4.53	5.44
Nutrient requirement			
DE (Kcal/kg diet)	3,550	2,785	2,360
DE (KJ/Kg diet)	14,840	11,648	9,885
ME (Kcal/kg diet)	3,400	2,670	2,270
ME (KJ/Kg diet)	14,250	11,182	9,490
CP (%)	22.7	15.2	14.0
Lysine (%)	0.91	0.75	0.81
Methionine (%)	0.70	0.47	0.53
Methionine + Cysteine (%)	1.04	0.75	0.77
Cysteine (%)	0.35	0.26	0.23
Threonine (%)	0.74	0.57	0.61
Tryptophan (%)	0.23	0.17	0.22

Source: Paul *et al.* (2007), NRC (1998), ARC (1981)

Table 9. Dietary requirements (as fed basis) of crossbred pigs having higher growth potential

Age (weeks)	8 to 16	17 to 24	25 to 32
Body weight (kg)	11.5 to 44	45 to 80	81 to 110
Av weight (kg)	27.675	61.737	95.119
BW gain (g/d)	577	640	553
Av daily feed intake (g/d)	1,550	2,400	3,360
Feed: Gain	2.70	3.74	6.07
Nutrient requirement			
DE (Kcal/kg diet)	3,685	3,185	2,125
DE (KJ/Kg diet)	15,417	13,328	8,890
ME (Kcal/kg diet)	3,537	3,058	2,040
ME (KJ/Kg diet)	14,801	12,795	8,535
CP (%)	21.4	16.5	12.6
Lysine (%)	0.70	0.79	0.73
Methionine (%)	0.66	0.51	0.48
Methionine + Cysteine (%)	0.34	0.28	0.20
Cysteine (%)	1.0	0.82	0.69
Threonine (%)	0.77	0.63	0.55
Tryptophan (%)	0.21	0.19	0.20
Calcium (%)	0.70	0.60	0.50
Phosphorus (%)	0.60	0.50	0.45
Av. Phosphorus (%)	0.30	0.25	0.20
Sodium (%)	0.14	0.11	0.11
Chloride (%)	0.14	0.10	0.10
Potassium (%)	0.26	0.22	0.20
Copper (mg/kg)	5.0	4.0	4.0
Manganese (mg/kg)	3.0	2.5	2.5
Iron (mg/kg)	70	60	50
Zinc (mg/kg)	70	60	55
Selenium (mg/kg)	0.20	0.16	0.16
Iodine (mg/kg)	0.15	0.15	0.15
Vitamin A (IU/kg)	2,000	1,600	1,500
Vitamin D (IU/kg)	200	160	150
Vitamin E (IU/kg)	15	12	12
Riboflavin (mg/kg)	3.0	2.5	2.2
Niacin (mg/kg)	12	10	8
Thiamin (mg/kg)	1.2	1.2	1.2
Pyridoxine (mg/kg)	1.5	1.2	1.2
Pantothenic acid (mg/kg)	9	8	8
Folic acid (mg/kg)	0.32	0.32	0.32
Biotin (mg/kg)	0.06	0.06	0.06
Vitamin B_{12} (mcg/kg)	15	10	7
Choline (mg/kg)	400	350	350

Source: Paul et al. (2007), NRC (1998), ARC (1981)

It may be concluded from the studies carried out in the last 50 years under AICRP on Pigs North-East Agricultural Research Complex of ICAR and under AP Cess Fund ad-hoc scheme of the ICAR on indigenous, exotic and crossbred are scanty, short term and since majority of the pigs in the country are raised under scavenging conditions or fed on waste human food and other crop and livestock wastes, with highly variable nutrient content and availability, it is extremely difficult to give any specific recommendation either on nutrient requirement or quantity of feed to be given. Most recommendations in the country have been made on the basis of short term feeding trials essentially using NRC/ ARC recommended feeding standards. Except for intensive rearing of pigs of defined genetic constitution and under standardized housing and health management, the standard recommended by ARC/ NRC or developed by various research organizations within the country can only be used as a guide and will have to be modified through further experimentations.

4.9 Formulation of economic rations for pigs

A ration is a feed allowance for an animal in quantitative and qualitative terms to be given in 24 hrs and meet the maintenance and production requirements. The nutritional requirement vary according to production type, breed within production type, sex, age and functional status. It must meet the energy (caloric requirement), protein (amino acids), vitamins and minerals. It must be palatable, energy dense so that the quantity consumed can meet the nutrient requirement. Ration can be offered once, twice and more time in a day. It is now a common practice to feed *ad lib* so as to maximize production without reducing the efficiency of feed conversion.

Ration formulation should involve achieving the best possible nutrient balance of key nutrients in a practical and financially viable manner. The ration formulation would have the following the priorities:

i) To deliver adequate quantity of different nutrients to meet the maintenance and production requirements.
ii) To optimize nutrient utilization.
iii) To reduce the cost of ration and maximize economic returns.
iv) To be fed effectively with the equipments and facilities available. The feed formulation does involve mathematical calculations of the

quantities of various ingredients to be combined. It should also consider the cost of the ingredients and alternate sources of nutrients available at a relatively cheaper price.

The considerations in ration formulation are:

i) Its palatability and intake with least refusal/leftover.

ii) The feeds should have higher digestibility and release the nutrients more efficiently in gastrointestinal tract of the animal. They do not have high fiber content which cannot be tolerated by swine.

iii) It has low cost but the cost should not compromise with the quality which determines intake and utilization thus the various functions related to production.

iv) It should not contain anti-nutritional factors and toxins. The anti-nutritional factors are ante-trypsin factor in soybean meal. Some ingredients may contain mycotoxin / aflatoxin beyond the tolerable limit.

v) High moisture content reduces keeping quality due to fungal infestation as well as reduces intake.

Since the feed accounts for the 55-70% of the cost of production, it would require serious attention to maximize the profitability (minimum on feed cost) in pig production. Proper analysis for nutrient composition of the various ingredients and their cost would decide their incorporation in the compounded feed. Further different functional groups and different stages of function would require feed with different levels of proportions of nutrients. It would require a scientific planning of least cost and most productive rations. Therefore to properly formulate a ration of a functional group of pigs, the following points should be considered.

i) The nutrient requirements for different production functions

ii) The feed ingredients available, their nutrient content, price and any incriminating factors present

iii) Quantity required per batch

iv) Techniques used in formulation of feed.

4.10 Nutrients requirements and limitation of nutrient availability

The primary concern is to formulate a ration to meet the nutrient requirements; however, some nutrients can create problems of intake and digestibility and may have poor efficiency of feed conversion. Such ingredients should be used at the lowest level.

4.11 Limitations in use of feed ingredients

After knowing/determining nutrient requirement, specific category of feed, ingredients may be selected. Feed ingredients can be divided based on specific functions such as an energy sources, a protein sources, a mineral sources, a vitamin sources and other feed additives. Grains are primarily energy sources, oilseeds/cakes/meals and slaughter waste by-products, fish meal are primarily protein sources. Common salt and mineral mixture and vitamin supplement are added to make the feed balanced. Maize is the traditional energy source in swine diets and soybean meal a primary source of protein, both have satisfactory digestion and efficient utilization.

4.12 Batch size

The feed compounded at a time to meet the nutrient requirement for the requisite number of animals and requisite number of days constitutes a batch and would vary according to the number of animals and storage capacity. Most commercial feed size are of 2-3 ton capacity and will store feed ingredients accordingly.

4.13 Diet formulation

Rations are formulated differently but the main objective is to provide a low cost balanced ration. This can be done by:

1. Square method which is relatively simple and satisfies only one nutrient requirement and uses only two feed ingredients. Another limitation is the level of nutrient being computed should be intermediate between the nutrient concentrations of the two feed ingredients being used.

2. Simultaneous equation method: It uses a simple algebraic equation working out a particular nutrient requirement using a combination of two feed ingredients.

3. Two x Two matrix method: This method forms two nutrient requirements using two different ingredients. A two x two matrix is set and a series of equation come up to find the solution to the problem.

4. Trial and Error method: This is the most popular method for formulating ration for swine and poultry. The formula is manipulated until the nutrient requirements are met with.

5. Linear Programming involves determining least cost combination of feed ingredients using a series of mathematical equations. This provides a number of possible solutions with the application of cost of compounded feed. Only the least cost formulation is selected. With the availability of electronic computer all the possible feed ingredients, their nutritional value and cost can be fed and various combination which meet nutritional requirements and have least cost are worked out. It should, however; be realized that least cost ration may not provide most economic animal performance. Further the least cost ration may have poor palatability and thus may not provide adequate intake. The keeping quality of the compounded feed arising from least cost formulation also needs to be considered.

4.14 Procedure for formulation of ration using linear programming

It would require the following steps:

1. Availability of feed ingredients,
2. Nutrient composition of feed ingredients,
3. Ration specifications,
4. Computer procedure that would meet the desired specification at the lowest possible cost. The calculation may involve an algebraic method.

❑❑❑

CHAPTER-5

Pig Diseases – Prevention and Control

Under extensive management conditions, pigs are exposed not only to environmental stresses and feed and nutrient inadequacies but are also affected by a large number of infectious and systemic diseases. There is little effort for provision of any prophylaxis in indigenous pigs managed extensively and only in case of extreme mortality or in zoonotic diseases some efforts for control and eradication is taken by the Animal Husbandry Department. Under the extensive and semi-extensive management conditions the pigs are exposed to bacterial, viral and parasitic diseases.

5.1 Bacterial Diseases

There are several bacterial diseases of pigs with varying incidence and resulting in variable economic losses due to mortality and morbidity. The diseases with significant impact on pig health and production and widely prevalent in India can be broadly classified in to (i) diseases affecting gastro-intestinal tract, (ii) diseases affecting respiratory tract, (iii) diseases having multi-systemic and (iv) other bacterial diseases.

5.1.1 Gastro-intestinal infection

5.1.1.1 Enteric colibacillosis

E.coli infection is common in the first week of life of piglets and again in the first week after weaning. It can also be secondary to other infections including rotavirus and urinary tract infection. Infection in neonatal piglets is common due to sudden exposure to bacterial infected skin of the mother and in farrowing environment. Diarrhea appears within 2-3 hours of infection. The faeces may be clear white or brown in color. In severe cases there is dehydration, mortality up to 70% can be observed.

5.1.1.2 Post-weaning E.coli

The infection reflects neonatal hygiene and infectious conditions, there is brownish diarrhea and dehydrated condition. There is a reduction in feed intake and in severe cases there is lethargy and disorientation. Mortality rate is low (10%).

The diagnosis is based on clinical symptoms and isolation of infecting agent. There are a large number of pathotypes. A large number of conventional and DNA based serotyping are now available.

The treatment involves administration of antibiotics but specificity of suitable antibiotics should be determined. Dehydration can be prevented through administration of glucose fluid. Proper management and provision of clean sties free from direct cold winds can reduce the incidence. Proper disinfection of the farrowing pen before farrowing can help in reducing the incidence.

5.1.1.3 Oedema

Oedema disease is a per-acute toximea caused by specific pathotype of *E.coli* that affects primarily healthy, rapidly growing, nursing pigs. It is also known as gut/ bowl oedema. In addition to the oedema, nervous signs and central nervous system lesions can be observed. The disease occurs within 10 days of weaning and affects the well grown piglets. Piglets become infected initially by a contaminated concentration of sow. Spread of infection among pen mates is facilitated by a large number of oedema disease producing *E. coli* that are shed by colonized pigs. High protein diet increases the susceptibility to the disease. Factors associated with weaning include the stresses of mixing with other piglets, changes in diet and loss of the milk antibodies from the intestine. Affected piglets appear dull, may appear blinds and may press their heads against hard surface. There is in-coordination and lack of balance. Clinical symptoms and detection of genes for VT II e through PCR can confirm the infection. The piglets which cannot walk after 3 days should be destroyed. Anti-microbial drugs are of little use. Prevention through proper hygiene is the only proper procedure.

5.1.1.4 Clostridial infection

Clostridium perfringens types A and C cause diarrhea, dysentery and death in pigs. The toxins of *C. perfringens* type A cause secretion of fluid in the small intestine, and some inflammation and diarrhea. It may also reach high numbers and cause diarrhea in the weaning pig. Disease in piglets is prevented by passive immunity from the colostrum of an immunized mother. Piglets affected by *C. perfringens* type C are generally born to sows without immunity, are normal at birth, sicken on the first or second day after birth and usually die within 12-24 hours of onset of clinical signs. Fatal bloodstained diarrhea in piglets of 36-48 hours of age strongly suggests *C. perfringens* type C infection. Oral ampicillin can be used to treat the survivors of an affected litter and given soon after birth, may prevent the occurrence of the disease completely.

5.1.1.5 Salmonellosis

The disease is caused by *S. enteric*. Pigs are affected easily between weaning and 3-4 months of age. They look depressed and dull with weakness and even may show nervous symptoms. Paralysis and trauma may also be observed. Clinical signs and isolation of infected agent or detection of virulence factors through PCR can be used. The affected animals may be treated with antibiotics. Use of clean and heat treated feed and water, rodent and fly control can help in reducing the incidence.

5.1.2 Diseases mostly involving respiratory tract

Respiratory diseases of pigs can be classified into two broad categories based on the extent and duration of the disease; which affect the large number of pigs and may be serious but persists for a limited duration, affects a large number of pigs for an indefinite period. Diseases in the first category can be costly for the losses in the limited time and include mostly viral diseases. In the second category, are diseases like mycoplasmal pneumonia, pluro-pneumonia and atrophic rhinitis. It is difficult to keep herds free from respiratory diseases. Aerosols have been suspected as a source of pathogen entry from the neighboring farms. Some of these infections can travel over miles depending on climate and intensity, and location of pigs in locality. Introduce new animals only after proper quarantine or use of AI/ ET for introducing superior germ plasm can avoid introduction of new infection or its variants. Multiple site production, all-in or all-out can help in minimizing the potential effect of chronic infection.

5.1.2.1 Atrophic Rhinitis

Progressive Atrophic Rhinitis (PAR) is caused by a strain of *Pasteurella multocida.* The clinical symptoms involve sneezing and snuffing in younger pigs accompanied with tear stained or bleeding eyes. Subsequently there is a displacement of jaw. Clinical signs, isolation and identification of the organism can confirm the diagnosis on the basis of clinical symptoms. A large number of modern molecular tools are now available for confirming the disease. Treatment with broad spectrum antibiotics can help.

5.1.2.2 Swine Erysipelas

It is caused by the bacterium *Erysipelothrix rhusiopathiae* and is very closely related to *E. tonsillarum.* The organism is localized in the skin, the joints or the heart valves and causes skin lesions, arthritis and endocarditis. The infection results in sudden death. After dullness and high temperature, a scarlet flush can be seen on the skin. Inappetence, high fever are common symptoms. There may be flushing, blotching of the skin and ears. Diamond shape skin lesions occur within 48 hours of the onset of clinical signs. The characteristics skin lesions can help in diagnosis. Culture examination of blood and postmortem examination of dead animals can help in confirming diagnosis. Treatment involves administration of antibiotics for 2-3 times daily.

5.1.2.3 Mycoplasma Arthritis

The disease is caused by *M. hyosynoviae* which can be distinguished from other mycoplasma by fermentation of arginine but not glucose and urea and by its antigen.

Few clinical signs occur. The animal may show lameness. Acute lameness in old fattened pigs or recently introduced breeding stock with no fever or evidence of polyserositis suggest the presence of the infection. Treatment in early clinical cases may involve taimulin @1.5mg/kg on 2-3 successive days.

5.2 Viral Diseases

5.2.1 Classical Swine Fever

It is caused by RNA pesti virus. The incubation period is 5-10 days. The young piglets die without showing any symptoms. In acute cases there is dullness, lethargy, loss of appetite and rise in temperature. This is followed by conjunctivitis and constipation followed by diarrhoea with occasional vomiting. Piglets hurdle together. There is a swing movement on the hind quarters making the animals to seek the wall, reddening and broaching of the skin and dypsnea occurs. Convulsions also occur in the early stages which are followed by circling, in-coordination and ataxia. The animal dies within 4-9 days of infection in hyper acute cases.

High fever in large number of animals along with dullness, lethargy, in-appetence and conjunctivitis are signs of the disease. Swing and seeking support of the walls and poles with high mortality show the possibility of swine fever. There is no treatment; however, protection through vaccination with live attenuated vaccine is possible.

5.2.2 Rotavirus infection

Groups A, B, C and D of the virus cause infections in pigs. Group A is generally first to infect and is most common infection in pre-weaning piglets. Incubation period averages between 18-24 hours and leads the diseased pig to depression, inappetence and reluctance to move. There may be diarrhea in suckling piglet which may be yellow or dark grey. There is no specific treatment. Feeding of cow's colostrum to sows during pregnancy can help in protecting against rotavirus. Proper cleaning and disinfection is required.

5.2.3 Transmissible Gastro-Enteritis (TGE)

The disease occurs as an explosive outbreak of diarrhea which involves pigs of all ages. The diarrohea is profuse, watery and yellowish green. It may have bad odour and contain undigested milk or floccules of curd. Vomiting may occur. The death takes place within 24-48 hours. The clinical signs with extensive incidence in deaths in young piglets and further pathological findings can confirm the disease. There is no treatment. The effected piglets can be given electrolyte.

5.2.4 Porcine Reproductive and Respiratory Syndrome (PRRS/ Blue Ear)

It is caused by arterivirus. The disease in sows and boars begin with inappetence lasting up to 4-7 days. Animal become restless, have labored breathing with rare rise in temperature. Reddening of skin, purple colouring of ears appears in 22 days. Antepartum deaths results in birth of a large number of mummified piglets. There is also an increase in mortality. Increase in still births up to 20%, abortions up to 8% and pre-weaning mortality up to 26% would cause suspicion of the disease. Virus isolation is the only confirmatory test. There is no specific treatment. Supportive measures can reduce losses and involve uses of aspirin for 7 days prior to farrowing which can provide some protection.

5.2.5 Foot and Mouth Disease (FMD)

FMD in pigs involves seven serotypes viz A,O,C, SAT-1, SAT-2, SAT-3 and Asia-1. Each type has several subtypes. The clinical signs involve severe lameness, arched back, reluctance to move and mostly lying down. Vesicles appear on the snout and on the udder of the suckling sows and may rupture readily leaving small ulcers. Clinical signs are severe lameness. The inspection of feet, snout and tongue of lame pig will confirm the disease. Piglets are not readily immunized as they require high concentration of virus. Immunity however has been demonstrated for about 9 months using oil adjuvant vaccine.

5.2.6 Swine Pox

It is caused by swine pox virus. The incubation period is 3-6 days which may go up to 14 days. As red one cm papules on the ventral abdomen later turning into circular and brown are observed. These scabs are later turn into black. The size, colour and circular shape of the lesions is characteristics of the disease. Treatment and control are rarely attempted because of mildness of the disease. Spread of this infection can help in reducing lice and flies which spread the disease.

5.3 Parasitic Diseases

The importance of internal and external parasites in pig production varies greatly among different geographical regions because of differences in topography, climatic condition and husbandry practices. Range managed pigs are exposed to greater parasitic infestations and there is a greater difficulty to control because of fast reinfection. They are also exposed to more inclement weather and poor nutrition. External parasites include mange mites, demodactic mites, lice, fleas, mosquitoes, flies and ticks, which can produce a range of clinical signs due to scratching, bites and resulting in skin lesions.

They cause serious economic loss due to reduced growth, reduced efficiency of feed conversion and loss of value of carcass at slaughter. Ectoparasites also contaminate the pork and act as vectors for microbial pathogens. Internal parasites are very common and impact production due to discomfort and interference with the consumption and utilization of feed and may cause clinical diseases. Some internal parasites are found in lungs and interfere with respiration and may cause pneumonia. Even though internal parasites are commonly associated with free range managed animals, they also affect intensively managed animals if proper hygiene is not maintained.

5.3.1 External parasites

5.3.1.1 Sarcoptic Mange (Scabies)

It is an important problem in swine worldwide. The scabies is caused by two types of parasites viz *Sarcoptes scabies* variety *suis and Demodax phylloides* or follicular mange which is less common. The animal suffering from scabies becomes irritable and uncomfortable because of intense itching. It depresses growth rate and feed efficiency, and further decreases fertility in breeding sows. The mites spread directly through contact with infected pigs.

Two clinical forms of the disease viz hyper-caratotic which affects mostly multi-parous sows and causes pruritics or hypersensitivity and further affects growing piglets. The boar helps in maintaining infection in the herd because of its contact with breeding sows and gilts at the time of mating. The infection is more common in group housed pigs. Environmental spread is less important especially if the pens are exposed to direct sun light. Proper disinfection can reduce the incidence of mites and thus the infection. Effective control is through vacating the shed and its proper disinfection.

The diagnosis can be confirmed by demonstration of the presence of the mites. Looking at the inside ears/ groin/anus can show the mites. A tea spoon is an ideal instrument for scratching the inside of the ear and spreading the material on the black paper and turning it upside down and only mites will continue sticking to the paper, they then can be examined under the microscope.

Treatment involves injection of Ivermactin. A single injection of 300 microgram per kg body weight given to sows 8 days before farrowing is very effective in preventing their transmission to piglets.

Segregation of affected animals, their proper treatment and removal of the bedding and spraying the premises with anti-parasitic agents can remove the infection.

5.3.1.2 Demodectic Mange

It is relatively unimportant in pigs because it affects the skin follicles. Transmission occurs through contact of neonates with nursing mother or through huddling. The Acarisides used for Sarcoptic mange can be used in this infection.

5.3.1.3 Lice

Lice are relatively uncommon in a pig herd particularly if mange is regularly treated as the treatment also kills lice. They cause irritation and suck blood but economic losses are relatively low although severe infestation can cause anemia. The lice affecting pig is *Haemopynus suis* and has piercing and sucking mouth parts. They are found on all parts of the body but particularly on folds of the skin around the neck, mouth and flanks and inner surface of the legs. Direct contact with affected animal results in the spread of disease. Treatment involves sprays, Ivermactin injections and medication through feed. Bedding can be sprinkled with insecticide granule.

5.3.1.4 Ring Worm

Fungal diseases tend to be superficial mycoses involving the keratinized epithelial cells and hair and are of little economic importance. It affects both animal reared indoor and outdoor and all age group, unhygienic conditions, high stocking rate with moderate temperature with high humidity provide conditions for spread of ringworms. The lesions start as circumscribed lesions which tend to circle and make on complete site of pig. The skin is light brown in colour, roughed but not raised. A brown crust may appear on the ear and neck. *Candid albicans* is the common cause of the disease in pigs. Treatment consists of removal of crust and local application of disinfectant or antiseptics. The house can be disinfected by phenolics or sodium hypochloride.

5.3.1.5 Ticks

Two kinds of ticks infest pigs viz hixodid (hard) and argasid (soft). Ticks can be readily seen through visual examination and can be present on any part of the body but more often around the ears, neck and flanks. Depending on the blood engorgement, the size of the lesions varies. They are responsible for transmission of protozoa, and viruses. The ticks commonly attack ears, neck and flanks. The treatment in pigs is rarely necessary as the few ticks present can be easily removed.

5.3.1.6 Mosquitoes and flies

Cause nuisance and are present due to unhygienic conditions. Proper sprays/fogging can reduce the presence and their nuisance to the animals and its possible spread of the disease.

5.3.2 Internal Parasites

5.3.2.1 Helminthes

5.3.2.1.1 Large round worm (Ascarids)

Ascaris swm, the large round worm is the most common nematode in the pigs especially up to 2-3 months of age. Sows are not affected but serve as carriers. The adults parasites live in small intestine ingesting particulate and liquid materials. The small larva penetrate the gut wall and are carried to the liver through the blood stream and may be subsequently taken to the lungs.

Clinical symptoms include inflammation of the liver, spots on the liver, thicken lung tissue leading to inefficient respiration and causing great pain. The worms compete with the animal for feed and reduce efficiency of feed conversion.

The presence of eggs does not help in diagnosis. The symptoms caused by the parasites and pathological lesions on postmortem can confirm the infection.

5.3.2.1.2 Whipworm-Trichuris suis

The parasite is found in caecum and upper and large intestine. It penetrated the gut lining, causing irritation and some blood loss. Blood tinged diarrhea may occur.

5.3.2.1.3 Nodular worms

Represent larval stage of *Oesophagostomum*. These nodules are formed by a fibrotic host response in the walls of the caecum and colon. Larvae that escape nodule formation emerge in the gut and mature in to adults. Condemnation of large intestine or colon at slaughter results in economic loss as these cannot be used as sauces casings. In adult pigs it can cause diarrhea.

5.3.2.1.4 Thread worms

Threadworms or strongyloides are seen in young piglets, living in the wall of small intestines. Farrowing pens, dirt lots and pastures get contaminated with larvae that hatch and may be ingested through feed and water or may penetrate skin. The infected larvae may also pass through sow colostrums and infect the piglets.

The infection results in intensive diarrhea in neonatal pigs causing dehydration. Protective immunity can be produced. Kidney worm, stephanurs is short stout black and white parasite found in the fat around the kidney and sometimes inside the kidney. Mature worms are found mostly in sows as it takes 9-12 months to reach adult stage. Wood logs and shaded farrowing pens often become contaminated with the larvae after hatching and the soil infective larvae or infected earthworms harboring the larvae can infect the pigs. From the liver, the larvae migrate to areas into the kidney and even into the back muscle. The liver and nearby muscle are most damaged.

5.3.2.1.5 Lungworm

Metastroglus are short, cylinder and white parasites occurring in cluster in respiratory tract (bronchioles). Eggs are coughed up, swallowed and pass in the faces. Lung worm eggs are ingested by earthworms which allow easy exposure to pigs as they root in the soil and eat infected earthworms. The larvae pass from the small intestine through the heart into the lungs resulting in thumping or coughing with pneumonia.

5.3.2.1.6 Coccidiosis

Isopora suis is responsible for coccidiosis in piglets which results in diarrhea. The clinical signs involve malabsorption of feed, diarrhea, loss of condition and some deaths. The faces may be whitish and firm and they may also be transient pasty diarrhea or profuse yellowish watery diarrhea between 5-15 days of age. There is a loss of condition. The occurrence of whitish, malabsorptive diarrhea in piglets is between 5-15 days of age. Oocytes can be seen in feces under light microscope.

The disease can be treated by trimethoprin/sulphonamide which should be supported by infusion of electrolyte.

❑❑❑

CHAPTER-6

Pig Reproduction

6.1 Male Reproduction

6.1.1 Techniques for semen evaluation, preservation and artificial insemination (AI)

AI enables a widespread use both spatially and temporarily of genetically superior breeding males in characters which have low heritability and expressed only in female such as litter size and mothering ability. Selection can be made only in the females on the basis of their own expression or the males on the basis of their dams, female collaterals and female progeny. To use such selected male extensively, AI can be very helpful. Crossing of breeds differing in size may not allow natural service to breed smaller females with larger males and AI is the only alternative. When new breeds are introduced with a relatively small breeding population, AI can help in a wider spread of superior male germ plasm. AI also prevents spread of sexually transmissible diseases. Sire can be tested more efficiently and their semen can be used more widely, spatially and temporally.

The selected boars need training for donating semen in artificial vagina. A dummy or a non-pregnant and non-estrus sow can be used for collection of semen. The boars can be kept separately from breeding female herd. The boar should be gently handled and brought to the dummy/non-estrus sow. The collector should reach the prepuce and massage it to stimulate pelvic thrusting and the erection of penis. Once the penis is protruded and fully extended, it should be directed towards the AV for collection of semen. The AV should have a temperature of 37 °C. The gel from the semen should be separated from the sperm containing liquor. The semen in boar is ejaculated in three phases viz. pre-sperm, sperm rich and post-sperm fraction. Pre-sperm fraction is watery, a copious discharge and is the largest component of the volume of ejaculate, the second fraction is rich in sperms and is generally used for insemination.

6.1.2 Preservation of fresh semen

The semen is evaluated for sperm concentration, sperm motility, morphology and percentage of live and dead and abnormal spermatozoa. Motility is determined through the use of light microscope. The sperm should show active movement.

6.1.3 Sperm morphology

Percentage of morphologically abnormal sperms impact fertility and should not exceed 6-10%.

6.1.4 Sperm concentration

Live sperms concentration is measured by hemocytometer. The concentration of sperms should also be high and is normally 6-10 x^{10} /cc.

Staining a drop of semen on a slide with eosin nigrosin stain and made into a thin smear is examined under a microscope. 200 spermatozoa are examined to determine the percentage of live and dead sperms. Counting of physically abnormal sperms is also done.

6.1.5 Live Intact Acrosomes

This is also determined through a stained smear using Nigrosin-Eeosine-Geimsa stain. 200 sperms are examined. The semen after its examination for sperm motility, sperm concentration and percentage of live and normal sperms is extended using different extenders. Generally GEP extender containing (3.50 g potassium sodium tartarate) 1.00g, sodium citrate di-hydrate 0.03g, sodium salt of EDTA 0.20g, triple glass distilled water up to 100ml. Streptopenicillin 160mg/100ml extender, Gentamycin sulphate 3.2 mg /100ml of extender are also added to the extender. The extender should have pH of 6.8. After properly mixing, the extender is sterilized by autoclaving at 15 lb pressure for 20 minutes and is kept in refrigerator at 5 °C. The extender is warmed at the time of dilution in a water bath at 37°C and antibiotics are added at the final stage.

For preservation, the semen should be extended in a ratio of 1:4, however; if the demand is more, it can have wider ratio but should contain 3 billion sperms / c.c. of diluted semen. The diluted semen is maintained at refrigerated temperature till its use.

Successful AI in swine is influenced by number of days when onset of heat after weaning occurs. Gilts and sows should be bred after 10-12 hours after they are found in standing heat

Gilts/sows are inseminated after 4 h from the time of exhibition of estrus and 12-16h thereafter. They will show the signs of estrus 21-22 days again if not conceived. Before insemination the vulva and the surrounding portion should be cleaned with single use damp cloth or tissue paper. After stimulation of the sow, the catheter should be inserted slowly directed upward and forward and finally rotated counter clock wise till a resistance is felt. KY jelly may be applied around the sponge part of the catheter for smooth insertion.

6.2 Female Reproduction

The sow is polytocus and has no seasonality of breeding. It comes in heat every 21 days. Proestrus lasts about two days, estrus about 2-3 days and metestrus for 1-2 days and diestrus for the remaining cycle. The corpus luteum (CL) functions for 16 days after ovulation. Ovulation occurs spontaneously 36-44h after the onset of estrus or shortly beyond midestrus. Pregnancy lasts 112-116 days depending upon the litter size and the age of the sow.

6.2.1 Puberty

Breed and sire progeny group, season of the year, exposure to boar, type of housing, degree of confinement, level of nutrition and general health determines the age at sexual maturity. The percentage of gilts showing normal estrus cycle by 9 months of age is lower for those gilts reaching breeding age during summer than those in during other season. This is observed both in confined and free range managed animals. Confinement also reduces the percentage of gilts showing estrus at 7-9 months of age.

As gilts approach puberty, exposure to mature boar will shorten the expression of estrus and show synchronization of estrus. Puberty is often delayed if the gilts are exposed to the boar at the age of 3-4 months. Under normal conditions of feeding and management have little effect on age on puberty. The breeding cycle of female pigs is around 21 days with a range of 18-24. Most gilts of exotic breeds start cycling between 170-220 days of age when they are of around 90 kg live weight. Age and not the weight limit puberty in modern breed/strains of pigs when are well fed during growing period. Puberty is affected by breed, sire progeny group within a breed, season and stocking density. Mixing gilts during transport can also stimulate the onset of estrus. Contact with boar can also stimulate initiation of first heat. The male effect works better when young females are kept separate from the boar and introduced to the boar when 160-175 days of age. Prolonged exposure to male also inhibits expression of estrus. In commercial pig production gilts are normally mated when they express 3rd heat or when they weight 118 kg in exotic breeds. In native pigs, the gilts/ sows express heat much earlier both in terms of age and live weight. This has been explained earlier in chapter 3 on pig management. The female cycles every 21 days and show signs of heat through swelling and reddening of vulva 2-6 days before expression of heat. There is mucus discharge from vulva, the ears may be held erect and may point backward. The animal in heat may show restlessness and may go off feed. There is sniffing of genital organs of the other animals by the guilt/sow in heat. There is arching of back, rigid standing and allow easy handling of the back. There may be typical squeaky grunt and the seeking of male or other sows. Standing heat is when the male is accepted easily and lasts for 48h with a range from 38-60 h. First heat is usually shorter in length. The sows have longer receptive period than gilts. There is wide variation in duration of estrus according to genetic constitution, season and management system. Ovulation occurs in the second half of the estrus. It may be desirable for better conception if the female is bred twice in the same cycle. The sows should be rebred after farrowing early to have more litters and thus more marketable piglets but it will depend on their condition.

6.2.2 Estrus and sexual behavior

Length of estrus is variable and may lasts only for 12 h in gilts and may go up to 60 h or more in sows. Since it is difficult to know the actual time of onset of estrus, the sows/ gilts are mated/ inseminated twice during the estrus. This improves conception rate. The females in heat should be inseminated 12h after the standing heat is observed and again 18-24h after the first insemination. Starting with day1-2 after mating, the sows produce and release the hormone progesterone which is responsible for maintenance of pregnancy. If pregnancy does not occur, prostaglandin F_2 alpha is secreted by the uterus causing the regression of CL and secretion of progesterone on around day 17 of the cycle and development and maturation of a new crop of the follicles takes place and the animal is set to come in heat again.

In large pig farms where there is seasonal requirement of piglets to be marketed for slaughter for internal consumption of pork or export of pork/its products/live animals, there is a need to breed a large number of females simultaneously. There may also be demand for commercial processing of pork and a large number of animals of a particular weight or age are required. The reproductive cycle in female pig involves follicle stimulating hormone (FSH) secreted by anterior pituitary gland and responsible for growth and development of ovarian follicles. Each maturing graffian follicle has a maturing ovum. As the graffian follicle matures, it secrete estrogen which is responsible for animal's expression of heat and showing interest in being bred. Luteinizing hormone (LH) initiates the release of the ova. It is also secreted by anterior pituitary gland. Once the ovum is released from the follicle, it remains in the fallopian tube and later descends into the horn of the uterus. The remaining cells of ruptured follicles continue to develop into corpus luteum (CL). The CL secretes progesterone which is responsible for maintenance of pregnancy. If the ova are fertilized and become viable embryos, they attach themselves to the uterine mucosa and provide a feed back to the CL that signals to produce progesterone which is required for maintenance of pregnancy. Prostaglandin are secreted by uterus and fulfills the two roles, first in case of non-fertilization of ova thus no embryo to attach to the uterine mucosa and after 14-17 days of estrus, the uterus secretes prostaglandin which causes CL to regress stopping the secretion of progesterone. The second role of prostaglandin is to initiate parturition. During pregnancy as the foetus reaches its maturity, the pregnancy concludes and the uterus secretes prostaglandin which results in regression of CL and stoppage of secretion of progesterone and thus cause parturition.

The normal estrus cycle can be altered through hormonal treatment. P.G.600 is a combination of serum gonadotropin (Pregnant Mare Serum Gonadotropin-PMGS) and chorionic gonadotropin (Human Chorionic Gonadotropin) PMS and HCG. PMGS and HCG mimics FSH and LH respectively. In mature pre-pubertal PG600 will initiate estrus in non-cycling pre-pubertal gilts that are reaching puberty. Depending on the management conditions, gilts will reach maturity around 170-175 days of age. These are however too young to bred and the first heat is allowed to be escaped and these animals are allowed to be bred on second or third heat. PG 600 is not effective in cycling gilts. If a gilt is actively cycling and the CLs have secreted progesterone or are in the initial stages of regression, PG 600 has no effect on initiation of follicle development or release of ova. PG600 is most effective in breeding sows with extended return to estrus.

Matrix is a 0.22 % altrenogest solution, a synthetic progesterone. Its administration causes progesterone level to increase which extends the time period of the next ovulation. When matrix is discontinued, the anterior pituitary gland will be signaled to secret FSH leading to maturation of graffin follicle and expression of estrus. The time period between discontinued matrix and expression of estrus is normally 5-7 days similar to the return of estrus in weaned sows. Matrix must be filled daily as otherwise there will be poor results. Matrix is only used in gilts.

Prostamate and lutalyse are products of various forms of the naturally occurring prostaglandin F_2 alpha. These two products are approved in swine. If only one of these products is administered at the appropriate dose between 21-42 days of gestation, it will induce abortion and re-absorption of the litter. So for synchronization of sows that are at different phases of their estrus cycle and need to be bred simultaneously must be brought in heat together.

After day 1 of gestation, prostaglandin F_2 alpha may be used to induce pheromone. This can help in causing a large number of litters to be born simultaneously and thus provide better care and management and raised for market when there is large demand. For inducing farrowing the prostaglandin should be administered not more than one day before the average herd gestational length i.e. around 115 days.

6.3 Neuroendocrine function during seasonal reproduction

Regulation of oestrus relies on innate circannual and circadian rhythm of animals. The term circum refers to a cycle that has a length of approximately one year and repeats every year. Circadian rhythm is roughly 24h cycle in the physiological process of mammals. The circadian rhythm or pineal rhythms during the day is mediating photoperiodic information to the neuroendocrine reproductive system in many seasonal breeding mammals. Both rhythms are endogenously generated although they can be modulated by external factors. Of these photoperiod being the most important with regard to seasonal breeding and conception and other factors acting as modulators. To be able to utilize the rhythm in the prevailing photoperiodism, a neuroendocrinological regulation plays its role.

6.4 Biosynthesis and metabolism of melatonin

The biosynthesis of melatonin is initiated by the uptake of the essential amino acid-tryptophan into pineal parenchymal cells. Tryptophan is least available of the essential amino acid of normal diet. It is converted to another amino acid 5-hydroxyl tryptophan through the action of the enzyme tryptophan hydroxylase than to 5-hydorxytrptamine (serotonin) by the enzyme aromatic amino acid de-carboxylase. Serotonin concentration is higher in the pineal than any other organ or any brain region. It exhibits a striking diurnal rhythm remaining at maximum level during the day light hours and falling by more than 80% soon after the onset of the darkness as the serotonin is converted into melatonin, 5-hydroxytrptophol and other methoxyindoles. The conversion of Serotonin to Melatonin involves two enzymes that are characteristics of the pineal gland-serotonin-N-acetyl transferase-SNAT which converts serotonin to N-acetyl serotonin and hydroxyindol-O-methyl transferase (HIOMT) which transfers a methyl group to S-adenosylmethionine to the 5-hydroxyl with the N-acetylserotonin. The activity of both the enzymes increase soon after the onset of sun set because of the enhanced release of norepinephrine from sympathetic neurons parenchymal cells. Another portion of serotonin liberated from pineal cell after the onset of the darkness is de-aminated by the enzyme monoamine oxidase (MAO) and then either oxidized to form 5-hydroxyindole or reduced to form 5-hydroxytryptophol. Both of these compounds are also substrates for HIOMT and can thus be converted in the pineal gland to 5-methoxyindole acetic acid and 5-methoxytryptophol. The level of the latter indole, like that of melatonin, rises markedly in the pineal gland with the onset of the darkness. Since 5-methoxytryptophol synthesis does not require the acetylation of serotonin, the nocturnal increase in pineal SNAT cannot be triggered that causes pineal methoxyindole levels to rise. More likely a single unexplained process, the intra-parenchymal release of stored pineal serotonin, which then becomes accessible to both SNAT and MAO. This process ultimately controls the rates at which all three major pineal methoxyindoles are synthesized and generates the nocturnal increase in pineal melatonin and 5-methoxytryptophol. The proportion of available serotonin acetylated at any particular time of day light depends on the relative of the pineal MOA at that time. The rates of methylation of all the three 5-hydroxyindoles formed from pineal serotonin depends on HIOMT activity.

6.5 Photoperiodism

Photoperiod is the day length which varies considerably between seasons and is dependent on the latitude and longitude of the location. It is the most important external regulating factor in seasonal breeders. In addition to photoperiodism, many other environmental and management practice such as social stress in intensively reared large herds/ flocks, levels of feeding, boar contact, environmental factors viz. temperature, humidity, solar radiation and wind velocity are known to adjust the manifestation of seasonal infertility. Seasonality in breeding is a characteristic of animals that inhibit the higher altitudes that is depending on the distance from the equator. This is due to large seasonal variation in hours of day light and feed availability. During evolution the animals have opted to use changing photoperiod as a signal to provide appropriate timing of breeding season. Photoperiod is very reliable signal of the season compared to ambient temperature which can vary considerably at a particular time of the year. The applicability of artificial lighting programme is good option for commercial piggeries. The circadian melatonin secretion can be entrained by artificial lightening. Pigs are able to respond within relatively short acclimatization period to abrupt and extreme changes in ambient lightening. Indeed pigs are able to respond immediately to extension of dark phase as demonstrated by entrained melatonin profiles after the change from the 8 h dark phase to 16 h dark phase and becomes difficult for pigs to adjust to a change in other direction i.e. short day to long day. Pig can be made to respond to simplifying lighting regimens, light intensity during the photophase, so that pigs can differentiate between dark and light phases. The high intensity needed for differentiation between photo and scotophase is much lower in pigs and as low intensity as 40 lx which is enough to entrain melatonin secretion so that high melatonin concentrations occur in the systemic circulation during the dark phase. The phenomenon does not occur in pigs located closed to equator as the differences in hours of day and night are not large as in temperate countries located away from equator where the physical environment viz. temperature, humidity and feed resources affect expression of oestrus and thus some decline in seasons with high temperature and intensive sunlight without any protection and proper feeding show decline in incidence of oestrus.

❑❑❑

CHAPTER-7

Heat Stress in Pigs, Its Effects and Amelioration Measures

Pigs have efficient feed conversion efficiency under thermo-neutral zone (TNZ). Beyond this zone, pigs exchange the body heat through conduction (mostly through body contact with floor), convection (from body surface) and latent heat (through evaporative water loss from lungs). They do not have functional sweat glands and thus pigs have a limited capacity to lose heat by water evaporation from the skin (cutaneous evaporative cooling and generally use panting, a respiratory evaporative cooling).

When the temperature falls below TNZ, heat production by pig will be increased through shivering, directing the ingested energy from productive functions into heat production (cold thermogenesis), modifying the behavioral manifestation etc. The feed intake increases, animal grows slowly and feed conversion efficiency lowers when the ambient temperature is less than TNZ.

Higher ambient temperature may cause rise in rectal temperature, decrease in voluntary feed intake and decreased thyroid hormone production. The decrease in thyroid hormone production may be an apparent effort by the pig to slow its metabolism and thus its heat production. Furthermore, the effects of high ambient temperature on pigs are expected to be more pronounced at high relative humidity (RH). The higher the humidity level in the air, the less effective is the process of evaporative cooling which may adversely affect the pig production.

In the scenario of climate change, when heat stress is expected to increase and availability of water is expected to be reduced, information on the interaction of pig with its physical environment will be helpful.

7.1 Heat Stress Markers in Pigs

7.1.1 Physiological responses

7.1.1.1 Sweating verses panting

There are several species differences in heat transfer mechanisms, especially in terms of heat loss. In pigs, rodents, and dogs, panting is the major mechanism by which heat is dissipated. Panting increases respiration rate and decreases tidal volume, which increases ventilation and evaporation in the oral cavity and esophagus. Other mammals such as horses and humans rely predominantly on cutaneous evaporative heat loss via sweating for cooling the core temperature. Sweating is a more effective mechanism of heat dissipation compared to panting because panting requires muscle contraction, which in itself produces heat. This has implications for certain species and their susceptibility to heat stress. Specifically, pigs have little to no functional sweat glands which means they rely almost entirely on panting for heat dissipation. Additionally, swine possess a substantial layer of subcutaneous adipose tissue, which acts as insulation. Collectively, pigs have a high heat production and greater capacity to store heat, even under thermos-neutral conditions. These mechanisms may help partly explain why pigs may be more susceptible to heat stress compared to other species of domestic animals.

Under normal physiological conditions metabolic heat production due to muscle contractions, biochemical reactions, ion pump activity, etc. is offset by the body's ability to dissipate heat by radiation, convection and conduction. Heat is normally transferred to the atmosphere when ambient temperatures are below normal body temperature (i.e. a temperature gradient exists), but when ambient temperatures exceed the body's thermal-neutral zone (i.e. a reverse energy gradient), the only heat-loss mechanism is evaporative cooling via sweating. Generally, heat can be absorbed from the environment (via conduction, convection, or radiation) or generated metabolically due to increased growth, feeding, lactation, and other functions. On the other hand, heat can be removed from the body in addition to radiation, conduction, convection, cutaneous evaporation by means of urination, defecation, and milk removal. These increments of heat gains/losses are balanced within an animal to maintain euthermia. Heat stress occurs when the body can no longer maintain thermoregulatory homeostasis.

Due to inadequate sweat glands, pigs depend on panting as their primary mechanism of heat dissipation, especially if they do not have access to a wallowing area. The normal body temperature of the pig is 39.2°C (102.5°F) and at ambient temperatures above 22°C heat stress indicators such as increased respiration rates, and rectal temperatures are observed.

The physiology of the pig makes it very susceptible to climatic conditions, particularly temperature. Thermal stress among other climatic variables is a major factor negatively affecting production and reproduction of domestic animal species. Adult pigs are more prone to heat stress than cold stress as they have a better mechanism for retaining heat, especially due to well developed subcutaneous fat cover. The pig possesses sweat glands only on the snout and it is unable to dissipate a large amount of heat by sweating. However, in young piglets, due to low subcutaneous fat and large body surface area in comparison to its body weight they are more prone for cold stress and their temperature requirements are different.

However, as the means of dissipating heat in the pig are not very efficient, particularly in the absence of the opportunity to wallow, it will soon reach an upper critical temperature. This is associated with hyperthermia and heat stress and the pig will die if the situation cannot be reversed.

7.1.1.2 Feed intake (FI)

Of greater interest in the tropics is the effect of rise in ambient temperature. When the environmental temperature approaches body temperature, the pig will attempt to increase evaporative heat loss by sweating (through its limited sweat glands), panting, postural and positional changes, and wallowing in water, mud or excrement. In addition, it will reduce its energy output by decreasing its feed intake.

Voluntary feed intake is influenced by a number of factors and is very sensitive to environmental conditions. Feed intake in lactating sows decreases when the temperature exceeds 22 °C. Heat stress also causes decrease in milk yield and body weight during lactation. Feed intake decreases up to 50% during heat stress and this is often considered as the primary reason for negative effects on its production parameters. This decrease in nutrient intake explains a majority of weight loss, or lack of weight gain observed in heat-stressed domestic animals (DAs). Pigs decrease feed intake to maintain thermoregulation as eating and the process of digestion, absorption and assimilation increases metabolic heat production. It is thought that reduced nutrient intake is an attempt to offset the effect of environmental heat.

Heat stress studies in pigs have not thoroughly differentiated between the direct and indirect effects (i.e. reduced feed intake - FI) of heat. The reduction in FI due to heat stress may be responsible for the decreased body weight gain in growing pigs. Heat stress directly and indirectly (via reduced feed intake) affects physiology, metabolism, and performance in growing pigs. Heat stress directly altered aspects of post-absorptive metabolism by increasing circulating insulin concentrations. This elevated insulin inhibited lipolysis (illustrated by reduced circulating NEFA levels) and increased lipogenesis (via FAS enzyme activity). An increased heat load also directly alters protein metabolism by increasing muscle proteolysis. The reasons behind these alterations in whole-body energetics are not clear, but likely represent an evolutionary adaptation for survival.

7.1.1.3 Blood Flow

Other physiological responses to heat stress include a redistribution of blood flow from the viscera to the skin to aid heat dissipation. Due to the need for heat dissipation as a cooling mechanism, the body re-routes blood to the surface of the skin. Heat stress causes reduced venous pressure, and reduced heart, liver, splanchnic and thoracic blood volume. This diversion of blood to the periphery is accompanied by an increased cardiac output and this causes decreased blood volume.

Evidence also indicates reduced blood flow to the gastrointestinal tract (GIT) during heat stress. Reduced GIT blood flow can cause tissue hypoxia which depletes ATP stores and can potentially cause intracellular acidosis and changes ion pump activity. Depletion of ATP and acidosis can jeopardize tight junctions of the intestinal epithelium and this can result in bacterial and associated endotoxins and pathogens translocation across the membrane and into blood circulation. Heat stress can also cause increased tight junction permeability by increasing oxidative stress, and membrane damage. The result of bacterial translocation can lead to severe illness, endotoxemia or death as septicemia is very difficult to treat.

7.1.1.4 Effects on metabolism

Metabolism is a series of coordinated enzymatic reactions that allow organisms to prioritize energy (ATP) production, growth and reproduction. Metabolism consists of both catabolism (break down) and anabolism (constructing new molecules). Under stress, basic strategies of catabolic metabolism are involved in the generation of ATP (energy), to generate reducing power, as well as generating building blocks for biosynthesis. The universal currency of energy is ATP, which has high phosphoryl-transfer potential and hydrolysis of ATP drives reactions forward. It is generated from the oxidation of various fuel molecules. In humans the most important metabolic pathways are: glycolysis, citric acid cycle, oxidative phosphorylation, pentose phosphate pathway, urea cycle, fatty acid â-oxidation, and gluconeogenesis.

Heat stress has been shown to alter metabolism in several different DA species. Despite marked reductions in nutrient intake and body weight loss, heat-stressed ruminants increased basal and circulating insulin concentrations, while failing to mobilize adipose tissue triglycerides despite being in a hyper-catabolic state. This is intriguing because insulin is a potent anabolic signal that is typically down regulated under catabolic conditions.

Heat-stressed animals are thought to be in a catabolic state as epinephrine and cortisol are both typically increased during HS. Changes in blood glucose vary depending on DA species, as well as timing and severity of HS. However, it appears as though blood glucose is increased acutely, and then over time as feed intake decreases, as do circulating glucose concentrations. Circulating glucose concentrations have been shown to decrease in heat-stressed pigs and cows. However, other studies in poultry, rabbits, and pigs have shown increases in circulating glucose levels during HS. Heat-stressed pigs also have increased circulating triglycerides and cholesterol.

7.1.1.4.1 Insulin

Studies on insulin and hyperthermia are relatively recent but demonstrate interesting and perplexing results. Heat stress affects the insulin response in an unique way compared to other types of physical stress. Under most stress conditions, catecholamine production (such as epinephrine) inhibits insulin release in order to increase gluconeogenesis / glycogenolysis (to provide glucose for extra-hepatic tissues), and adipose tissue lipolysis (to provide fatty acids for skeletal muscle) to meet energy requirements. However, during a stressful heat-load, insulin is actually increased in most DA species, including a model of porcine malignant hyperthermia, rodents, and cows; despite a decrease in feed intake, reduction in blood glucose, loss of body weight and decrease in a calculated energy balance. In addition, the insulin response to a glucose bolus during heat stress is not altered compared to a thermal-neutral environment. Glucagon is also decreased in malignant hyperthermic pigs and this also leads to decreased availability of glucose and lipids for energy production.

7.1.1.4.2 Glucose metabolism

Heat-stroke patients often experience hyperglycemia which could indicate an increase in glucose production, or a decrease in tissue uptake. This has also been observed in a porcine model of terminal heat stress. The increase in production may come from an increase in glycogenolysis and/or gluconeogenesis. It has been demonstrated that during an increased heat-load, dietary carbohydrates are not able to reduce glucose production by the liver and hepatic glucose production increases. An increase in glycogen utilization may be due to enhanced anaerobic metabolism as lactate accumulation occurs in the muscle of heat-stressed humans. Heat stress effects on blood glucose are not entirely conclusive as decreases in blood glucose levels have been observed in different DA species including rats and ruminants. The reasons for the inconsistencies may be due to the type of experimental model, plane of nutrition, and timing/severity of heat stress.

7.1.1.4.3 Lipid metabolism

Stress hormones such as epinephrine normally induce lipolysis and increase circulating non-esterified fatty acids (NEFA) concentrations. Catecholamines are lipolytic and also inhibit insulin. However, during heat stress, mobilization of adipose tissue is not observed in a number of DA species including malignant hyperthermic pigs, cows and rodents. In a porcine model of terminal heat stress, animals exhibited an increase in NEFA concentrations; however this model represented a severely acute bout of heat stress. Heat stress also decreases fatty acid oxidation in humans. A heat load seems to favor retention of body fat as heat-stressed piglets have a greater percentage of body fat compared to piglets in thermal neutral conditions. It is interesting to note the relationship between carbohydrate and lipid metabolism during heat stress. Oxidizing fatty acids are less efficient in producing ATP (~13% less) than that of glucose which may help explain why more carbohydrates are utilized and adipose tissue is not mobilized during a heat-load.

7.1.1.4.4 Protein metabolism

Protein metabolism is affected by heat stress as muscle breakdown may occur. Tissue break down causes an increase in blood urea nitrogen (BUN) levels and this is often used as an indicator of muscle catabolism. Other indicators of muscle breakdown include increased plasma Nt-methylhistidine, creatinine, and creatine. Increases in these parameters have been observed previously during a heat-load in humans, chickens, and cows. Heat-stressed pigs also have an increase in plasma creatine kinase (CK) which is a measure of protein breakdown as it converts creatine and ATP to phosphocreatine and ADP. As insulin promotes protein accretion, it is interesting that protein catabolism is increased during a heat-load. Reasons for this are not clear however some hypothesize that protein is broken down in order for the liver to utilize the carbon in amino acids for gluconeogenesis.

7.1.1.5 Heat stress effects on cytokines

Cytokines are chemical messengers primarily released by macrophages, T and B cells, as well as other immune cells. These messengers can be either pro- or anti- inflammatory, and both types may be activated in the presence of heat-stroke. Bacterial infections, as well as heat stress or other types of physiological stress can induce cytokine release. A few major cytokines found to be associated with heat-stroke are: IL-1â, IL- 6, IL-10, IFNã, and TNFá. These cytokines are commonly elevated in patients admitted to hospitals with heat-stroke symptoms. Increased concentrations of IL-6 tend to be correlated with elevated mortality rates and IFNã in serum is increased in over 50% of heat-stroke patients.

Heat stress and reduced feed intake also causes alterations in intestinal barrier function, and can lead to "leaky gut". Increased permeability occurs due to elevated nitric oxide levels induced by cytokine stimulation. The "leaky" gut leads to an increased endotoxin concentrations in the blood and this elicits an immune response, thus releasing cytokines. These cytokines induce fever, or may actually cause hypothermia in the CNS. In the periphery, cytokine release causes systemic inflammation, leading to multi-organ damage, organ failure, and ultimately death.

Therefore, these sepsis and inflammation markers may also alter metabolism and nutrient partitioning and may explain why heat-stressed DAs have decreased production.

7.1.1.6 Heat shock response

Heat stress evokes a rapid heat shock response involving the activation of heat shock proteins (HSP). Heat shock proteins are a large family of stress proteins that are highly conserved across species and are aptly named according to their molecular weight. Their sizes and functions cover a wide range, but they generally serve as molecular chaperones or stabilizers of protein denaturation. These proteins can be increased due to heat, hypoxia, oxidative, and nutritional stress. Their activity is prevalent within several hours of the onset of severe stress and lasts for a few days. Expression of these proteins is mediated by activation of heat shock factor 1 (HSF 1). Heat shock factor 1 is a transcription factor, which binds to heat shock elements (HSEs) and initiates transcription of several heat shock genes.

One of the major inducible HSP family members is HSP70-72 kDa, which participates in protein folding, ubiquination, renaturing proteins, and providing protection during times of cellular stress. Heat shock protein 70 has also been shown to regulate toll like receptor (TLR)-4 signaling at the level of the intestine by targeting TLR-4 for degradation and subsequently diminishing the immune response.

Another important HSP include HSP 25/27, which is involved in thermal tolerance and protein ubiquitination (which targets proteins for degradation). Heat Shock Protein 25/27 is also an inducible protein, which helps maintain cytoskeletal structure, and protects cell architecture during stress. Studies in renal epithelial cells have shown that HSP 25/27 co-localizes with proteins in the actin cytoskeleton. In the intestine, HSP 70 and HSP 25/27 are integral in protecting the mucosal barrier under both normal physiologic, patho-physiological and stressful conditions. These are most abundant in the lower small intestine as well as stomach and large intestine.

Most of the biological function of HSPs occur in the cytosol. However, HSPs are also found extracellular and in the mitochondria. Traditionally HSPs were thought to be located exclusively in intracellular compartments of the cell. However, a little over 10 years ago researchers showed that HSP 70 was released into circulation after tissue necrosis and was involved in the immune response. Other HSPs such as HSP A5, HSP A9, HSP 60 and HSP 90 have also been found in extracellular spaces. Export of HSPs from the cell may primarily be a result of necrosis, or by a secondary type of unconventional secretary, active transport mechanism, or lysosome-endosome pathway. However, the mechanism by which HSPs are exported remains unclear and needs further investigation.

7.1.1.7 Hypoxia in heat stress

Heat stress induces hypoxia in visceral organs due to changes in blood flow and oxygen supply. Hypoxia is a condition within the body where the body is deprived of adequate oxygen supply.

7.1.1.8 Oxidative stress and heat stress

Reactive oxygen species (ROS) such as superoxide anion (O_2 -), hydrogen peroxide (H_2O_2), and hydroxyl radical (HO•) are produced during normal cellular metabolism, however during times of excessive ROS production, they can modify lipids, protein and DNA. Excessive ROS production is often termed "oxidative stress" and this can contribute to many types of pathological conditions. Mitochondria serve as an important source of ROS via the leaking or uncoupling of electrons from the electron transport chain. These free electrons then bind to molecular oxygen (O_2) to form superoxide (O_2•-), which is produced by reduction. These ROS bind to lipids, proteins and DNA and can damage the mitochondria themselves, or other organelles within the cell. Under normal circumstances, ROS are quickly dismutated by mitochondrial superoxide dismutase (Mn-SOD) to form H_2O_2. Mitochondrial electron leakage has been associated with the aging process, as well as several diseases including Parkinson's. In DAs, ROS production from the mitochondria has been shown to increase skeletal muscle protein degradation and reduced feed efficiency.

Antioxidants serve to combat the effects of ROS and maintain homeostatic redox balance within the body. Some major antioxidants of interest are various forms of superoxide dismutase (SOD), catalase, glutathione peroxidase (GSH-Px), glutathione transferase (GST), and heme oxygenase-1 (HO-1). These are all enzymes produced naturally in the body to scavenge free radicals. Some external or non-enzymatic sources of antioxidants include vitamin A, vitamin C, vitamin E, glutathione, and â-carotene.

7.2 Influence of Temperature and Humidity Stress on Reproduction in Pigs

7.2.1 Boars

Pigs have a low capacity for increased heat evaporation through sweating when the ambient temperature increases e.g. from 23 to

34°C, which contributes to the close relationship between environmental temperature and scrotal and testicular temperatures. Lowered fertility and lowered total sperm counts (TSC) and decreased ejaculate volume have been found in boars during or shortly after the warm summer period in several countries with temperate areas. In tropical areas, temperature has a significant negative effect on both the ejaculate volume, TSC and the morphology of the spermatozoa. A new housing system, called an evaporative cooling system (EVAP) or tunnel ventilation, has been introduced to improve the microclimate for DA production in regions with hot climate, in recent years. The EVAP system is a closed housing system, which aims to reduce the temperature via humidification process.

In a comprehensive Swedish/Thai study sperm production and sperm morphology was recorded in boars kept in EVAP system vs conventional housing system (CONV). Temperature and humidity were recorded on a daily basis during one calendar year. There was a higher diurnal variation and range over the year for both temperature and humidity in the CONV system compared to the EVAP system. The average maximum temperature was lower and the average minimum humidity was higher in the EVAP system, than in the CONV system. There was no overall difference in sperm production and sperm morphology between boars kept in the CONV and the EVAP housing systems. However, during parts of the year, differences between systems in sperm production and sperm morphology were observed. Elevated temperature had a significant negative effect on both the ejaculate volume and TSC in both housing systems. Elevated humidity had a significant negative effect on both the ejaculate volume and TSC in the EVAP system. To further minimize the negative impact of high temperature and high humidity on sperm production of boars under tropical conditions, further investigations on economically competitive technologies that can decrease both temperature and humidity are needed. In several experiments the effect of elevated temperature (in terms of heat stress) on the spermatogenesis of boars has been investigated using a climatic chamber.

7.2.2 Gilts and sows

Heat stress has been reported to reduce implantation and impair embryo development in pig. Gilts are more sensitive to heat stress before day 15 of pregnancy, than during days 15–30 post-breeding. A greater reduction in the number of viable embryos among gilts exposed to elevated temperatures during days 8–16 post-breeding than days 0–8 have been indicated that the time of implantation would be the most sensitive stage of pregnancy to stress. High ambient temperature leading to heat stress has been associated with seasonal infertility. This is especially true not only in tropical areas, where the temperature exceeds 30°C for several months of the year, but also in temperate areas. There has been a significant influence by climate, maximum temperature and heat index on litter size, farrowing rate and weaning to first service interval.

The management procedures in modern pig production include a number of events, which might act as stressors on the animals, e.g. high stocking densities, barren environments, transportation, poor or aggressive human-animal interactions and heat stress. Due to welfare consideration, systems with loose-housed sows instead of system with crates/stalls for the sows have become common, at least for non-lactating sows. These systems have several advantages: i.e. the animals have possibility to perform their natural behavior. However, there are factors in these systems causing problems. In systems with loose housed sows, the number of sows are in most cases much higher than in groups formed in the wild. The female pigs form family units of one or several sows and their offspring and the individuals in the family unit avoid contact with other unfamiliar sows. Therefore, in wild pigs (*Sus scrofa*) confrontation between unfamiliar female pigs happens very rarely. In commercial group housing systems, however, mixing of unfamiliar sows is difficult to avoid. A drawback with the group-housing system is also the difficulty to avoid regrouping. In most lactation units the sows are housed individually, and grouping of unfamiliar sows usually takes place at least once after weaning. A new social grouping in a limited space results in aggressive behavior among the animals. Depending on the social status of the animal, i.e. dominant or subordinate, different individuals have various capabilities in competing situations such as feeding and watering. An animal that does not cope with these situations may have a reduced health and production and also impaired reproductive performance. High ranked sows in oestrus will also mount submissive sows, and will increase stress. Elevated stress levels in a newly formed small group of sows may persist for approximately two days until a ranking order is established among the animals, and even continue for additional 10–12 days in large groups of sows.

The effects of stress on reproduction depend on the critical timing of stress, the genetic predisposition to stress, and the type of stress.

The effect of stress on reproduction is also influenced by the duration of the responses induced by various stressors. Prolonged or chronic stress usually results in inhibition of reproduction, while the effects of transient or acute stress in certain cases is stimulatory (e.g. in case anoestrus), but in most cases there is impairment in reproduction. Most sensitive of the reproductive process are ovulation, expression of sexual behavior and implantation of the embryo, since they are directly controlled by the neuroendocrine system.

7.3 Dietary Supplementation as Ameliorative Measures in Heat Stress

7.3.1 Glutamine

As heat stress has direct health implications to both humans and DA species, there is an interest in feed supplements as a way to improve the response to heat stress. Dietary supplementation is just one example of an easily adjustable and affordable option to be utilized in DA production and the biomedical field. In cattle, glutamine has been shown to enhance the immune response during heat stress by increasing IgG levels and lowering circulating concentrations of IL-6, and cows fed glutamine had a higher cell-mediated immune response than controls. Glutamine improves disruption of intestinal integrity as a result of ethanol and is associated with increased expression of HSP 70 and HSF-1. It has also been shown to prevent apoptosis in intestinal epithelial cells, decrease gut permeability and improve survival following environmental hyperthermia. Glutamine is a primary fuel source for enterocytes.

7.3.2 Zinc

Zinc has been shown to be essential for normal intestinal barrier function and regeneration of intestinal epithelial cells. It has been shown to improve intestinal integrity during malnutrition, ethanol-induced intestinal injury, inflammatory bowel disease as well as infectious diarrhea.

7.3.3 Chromium

Chromium may also be an option during HS. It facilitates insulin action on metabolism and as many studies have demonstrated, insulin is higher in heat-stressed animals, which may be part of a survival mechanism.

❑❑❑

CHAPTER-8

Pork, Its Characteristics and Processing

Pork specifically denotes fresh meat of the pig but it is wrongly used for all meats and meat products from pig which include cured, smoked or processed meat such as ham, bacon, and sauces etc. It is one of the most commonly consumed meat worldwide and more particularly in European countries. It is also the most common meat consumed in the North-Eastern region of India with a large tribal population. It accounts for 38% of the meat produced in the world. Although consumption of pork and pork products varies widely from country to country, it is becoming increasingly popular meat throughout the western world because beef and mutton have a higher fat content and thus have ill effects on the health of the consumers. Pork is consumed as cooked, cured or smoked or a combination of these methods. It is also consumed as an ingredient of sauces.

8.1 Chemical composition

Protein accounts for 19-23% of skeletal muscle and is grouped into three major categories viz. sarcoplasmic, myofibrillar and connective tissue proteins. Sarcoplasmic proteins are water soluble and can be extracted with salt solutions of lower strength such as 0.06m salt solution and accounts for 5-6% of the total muscle protein. It includes hemoglobin, myoglobin, cytochromes, flavoproteins, enzymes associated with glycolysis, tricarboxilic acid cycle and electron transport chain. Myofibrillar proteins also known as salt soluble proteins require higher concentration of salt for their extraction such as 0.3m salt solution and accounts for 11-12% of total muscle protein. It includes more than 20 different proteins falling in three different categories viz. contractile, regulatory and cytoskeletal proteins. The major proteins are myosin (45%), actin (20%), troponin (5%), tropomyosin (5%), titin (10%) and nebulin (4%). Connective tissue proteins also known as stromal proteins include insoluble fraction of proteins. Collagen, a glycoprotein is a major connective tissue protein which is a dominant protein in the animal body (20-25%) of the total body protein. Collagen has typical triple helix structure and is composed of three alpha chains of tropocollagan molecules. Elastin, a rubbery protein is mainly present in ligamentum nuchae and is highly insoluble in nature. A third type of connective tissue protein, reticulin was earlier regarded as a distinct protein but now-a-days it is considered as collagenous protein.

8.2 Fatty acid composition of pork muscle

Intramuscular fat varies from adipose fat where triglycerides constitute more than 99% of the total fat. Muscle fat has considerable amount of phospholipids and unsaponifiable constituents such as cholesterol in addition to triglycerides. Major fatty acids in muscle are palmitic, steric, oleic, linoleic and linolenic. Triglycerides also known as Neural lipids, have three fatty acids molecules (two in α position and one in β-position), esterifies to a glycerol molecule. Pig fat is peculiar in which the outer α-positions are occupied by unsaturated fatty acids which in most other species have these positions are occupied by unsaturated fatty acids. Phospholipids include phosphoglycerides, plasmalogens and sphingomyelins and are more complex than triglycerides. Phosphoglycerides include phosphatidyl choline, phosphatidyl ethanolamine, Phosphatidyal inositol and phosphatidyal serine. Sphingomyelin constitute about 10% of the phospholipids in which alcohol spingosine is bound by an amide link to a fatty acid and by an ester linked to phosphoryl choline. In plasmanogens, the second -OH group of glycerol is esterified with a long chain fatty aldehyde instead of fatty acid. The subcutaneous fat contains traces of lauric acid, 1-1.5% myristic, 25-30% palmitic, 10-14% stearic, traces of arachidonic acid, 2-4%, palmitooleic, 45-50% oleic acid, 5-7% linoleic acid and 0.1-0.3% linolenic acid.

8.3 Nutritive value of pork

The nutritive value of pork is attributed to its fats, carbohydrates, proteins, vitamins and minerals. Pork is a good source of essential amino acids and minerals. As the glycogen is converted into lactic acid during postmortem, the energy value of pork mainly comes from proteins and fat. Pork also contains a large amount of polyunsaturated fatty acids.

8.3.1 Proteins

Proteins account for 19-23% in raw meat and 25-30% in cooked meat. These proteins have high biological values i.e. it contains all essential amino acids in amounts equivalent to human requirement with high (95%) and easy absorbability. Among the essential amino acids, lysine and leucine accounts for about 8.5% each on the crude protein while tryptophan accounts only 1%.

8.3.2 Lipids

Constitute the most variable component. Pork is characterized by the presence of abundant subcutaneous fat which is generally lacking in other DA species. Intramuscular fat accounts for 4.4% in pork which is higher than the beef and kine (the buffalo meat) but has lower fat than the mutton. In general, the pork contains more than 50% of the unsaturated fatty acids mainly attributed to higher amounts of linoleic and oleic acid. It is rich in essential fatty acids viz, linoleic, linolenic, and arachidonic acids, each represents 2.0, 1.5 and 1.0 percent respectively of the total fatty acids. The cholesterol content in pork accounts for about 6 mg /100 g meat.

8.3.3 Minerals

Potassium is the most abundant in pork (350mg/100g) followed by phosphorus (275mg/100g). Other important minerals are sodium, magnesium, zinc, iron and copper in the descending order. It is deficient in calcium.

8.3.4 Vitamins

Lean pork has low vitamin contents. Liver is a rich source of vitamins. Pork is a rich source of thiamine (1IU/100g) compared to beef and chicken (0.1 IU/100g). The other vitamins present are folic acid (3 IU/100g), niacin (5 IU/100g), riboflavin, biotin, pantothenic acid, Vitamin B12, Vitamin B6 and traces of Vitamin A and D while Vitamin C is completely absent.

8.4 Simple methods for distinguishing pork from other meats

The pork can be distinguished on the basis of physical characters viz. appearance. It is grayish pink in color and has urine like odor. The fat is white, soft and characteristic subcutaneous fat deposit.

Chemically, intramuscular fat is 4.4%, myoglobin content 8-12 mg/g, iodine number of fat is more than 45.

Anatomically the pig has 45 % meat, 12-20% bone in carcass and 14-15% ribs.

Histologically the average muscle fiber diameter is higher in case of pork.

Although no single criterion can differentiate pork from other meats, a combination of physical, chemical and anatomical method can have a moderate to high reliability.

8.5 Factors influencing hygienic pork production

Farm to fork concept with proper hygiene which may involve pre-slaughter, slaughter and post slaughter hygienic handling can provide healthy pork.

8.5.1 Pre-slaughter factors

The importance of proper management of animals which involve the breed, selection methods for improving pork production and quality, nutrition, management and health affect pork production and quality. Improved pre-slaughter handling, proper drug administration, ensuring proper withdrawal period and ante-mortem examination can help in assuring proper quality of pork. These include:

i) Health care which involves proper administration of drugs especially antimicrobials, at a proper place and ensuring withdrawal at an appropriate time before slaughter.

ii) The pigs should not be exposed to stress during loading, transportation and unloading operations. These stress factors in addition to causing considerable deterioration, also cause easy transmission of microbes to the muscles. Feed withdrawal 12 h prior to slaughter thus facilitates in minimizing the ingested bacteria from the GI tract into blood stream.

iii) Anti-mortem examination of pig awaiting slaughter is necessary for hygienic pork production and safeguarding the health of the consumers. It should be conducted 12-24h prior to slaughter by a qualified veterinarian. The animals should also be examined before slaughter if the earlier examination was conducted 24h back. The ante-mortem examination should be able to detect if animal is suffering from any scheduled diseases communicable to human and could also be detected during postmortem examination. The postmortem examination is not only important for the health of the consumers but also for the health of the butchers and meat packers.

Anti-mortem examination is usually carried out at two stages viz. external examination before slaughter which involve general behavior i.e. posture and symptoms of any disease, and at the second stage; the temperature, pulse and respiration rate are recorded. The norms are 101°F, 75/min and 10-16/min respectively. The animals on anti-mortem examination may be classed as fit for slaughter, unfit for slaughter and suspect. In case of suspect, the animal can be held and re-examined after 24 h.

8.5.2 Slaughter practice

How the animal is handled at slaughter will determine the meat quality. The following steps are involved in slaughter of animals:

i) Stunning/immobilization which may involve mechanical stunning, which is least efficient in pigs.

ii) Bleeding- a 6" knife should be inserted mid way on the sternum to the throatlatch to accomplish free bleeding. The knife should be inserted with the point first directed upward and then moved downwards until it reaches vertebral column. With this incision, the carotid artery and jugular vein and even possibly the anterior vena cava are severed.

iii) Scalding and dehairing is done either by immersing the pig carcass in scalding. Pig containing water heated up to 60 °C until the hair/ scales begin to slip from the flank area. Hot water converts the collagen that surrounds the hair follicle into gelatin so that the hair can be removed either manually by scraping with a knife or using a dehairing machine.

iv) The viscera are then removed from the abdominal cavity and the pluck (lungs and heart) from the thoracic cavity. Anus must be cut loose from the attachment under the tail and the head is removed at the occipito-atlantal space. A cut is then made from the crouch to the sternum avoiding cutting the viscera or pluck. The carcass is then split down through the vertebral column. The carcass is then washed. The neck is trimmed of blood clots to ensure hygiene.

8.5.3 Post slaughter handling

It involves the important considerations necessary for hygienic pork production. It requires postpartum examination and proper post-slaughter handling. Postmortem inspection is necessary for wholesome pork production because a number of diseases and anatomical abnormalities are not detected during anti-mortem examination. The post-mortem examination should be done as soon as possible after dressing, as setting of carcass may render it difficult to examine its lymph nodes. Post-mortem examination includes the visual examination, palpation of organs and incision in them, if required. Regular laboratory test for confirmation may be required and should be carried through examination of lymph nodes as these nodes drain different parts of the body and the condition of a specific node would reflect the health of the part it drains.

Postmortem examination includes examination of carcass, fat and viscera. These may lead to a judgment viz. pass for human consumption, total condemnation, partial condemnation and conditional pass.

After slaughter, the handling of the carcass affects its hygienic quality. Extent of handling, quality of water used for washing carcass, hygienic condition of contact surface, knives etc. and the health of the butcher's and their hygienic handling of the carcass, packaging and dispatch including protection from flies and dust are factors that are important to be considered for ensuring for hygienic pork production.

Therefore, to ensure hygienic pork production, availability of appropriate premises for slaughter including ante and post-mortem examination, carcasses handling, packaging of meat and transport to destination. If the meat is not properly handled, not only it will lose its quality, but may get infected with pathogens which may result in spoilage of meat and cause health hazards to the handlers and consumers.

❑❑❑

CHAPTER-9

Bio-security Measures in Pig Production

9.1 Introduction

Currently pig production in the country is essentially an extensive backyard raising of a few piglets for sale for slaughter when there is a demand. Such pigs obtain their feed primarily from scavenging on household and human wastes. Such feed resources have a large risk of causing diseases to pigs which may have effect on the health of the pigs and thus the quality of the meat and a possibility of transmission of zoonotic diseases in human beings. In most countries, a variety of different pig production systems exist, from the simplest, with minimal investment, to large-scale market-oriented enterprises keeping pigs under intensive and comfortable management.

Raising scavenging pigs is the most basic traditional system of keeping pigs and the one most commonly reported in both urban and rural areas in most of the developing countries developing countries. In this free-range system, pigs roam freely around the household and surrounding area, scavenging and feeding in the street, from garbage dumps or from neighboring land or forests around villages. Very few arrangements are made to provide the pigs with housing. Depending on the local situation, pigs may be free-ranging for most of the year and penned during the rainy season. They may be housed at night in a small shelter, to protect them against theft and predators. Keeping scavenging pigs requires minimal inputs and low investment of labor, with no or limited money invested in concentrated feed or vaccines.

Small-scale confined pig production is also becoming common in developing and transition countries. Pigs are confined to a shelter, which can range from a simple pen made with local materials to more modern housing. The pigs are completely dependent on their keeper for feed, and receive tree leaves, crop residues, agricultural by-products or prepared feed. Smallholders raise pigs for both subsistence and commercial purposes. Pork is supplied to local markets and to more distant urban markets, through a complex marketing and transport system. Within this system, the financial risks for the producer can be high and there is limited support from organizations and professional bodies for technical inputs or services such as insurance.

The commercial farms under large-scale confined pig production system vary in size. Because consumers seek to purchase food at the lowest price, but the price of inputs is rising, the profit margin per pig is decreasing. Producers participating in global commodity pork markets must continually reduce the cost of production per pig to be profitable. Production can be on one site only or on several sites that are all part of the same structure. The major cost reduction measures that can be implemented when moving from small-scale to large-scale confined production are through increased farm size, specialization of farming activities, consolidation of the different steps of pig production, and adoption of an "all-in-all-out" production flow at each site, with implementation of some or even extensive bio-security protocols. Large pig farms may be family-owned, affiliated to companies or corporately owned.

In large-scale outdoor pig production, animals are confined by fencing, but are mainly outdoors; there is therefore less need for investment in bricks and mortar facilities. These farms can brand and sell pork for higher prices, and will often have a larger portfolio of activities, including agro-tourism or hunting for example.

Pig production is now being taken in an intensive and semi-intensive manner in urban and peri-urban areas utilizing various human food wastes, vegetables, meat and other food processing by-products which are usually not utilized as human food.

The extensive nature of management and thus exposure to inclement weather and poor and unhealthy feed resources create serious bio-security problems to pigs and transmission of zoonotic diseases to man.

Bio-security and earlier bio-safety has been considered important in raising meat animals. Bio-security is defined "the implementation of measures that reduce the risk of the introduction and spread of disease agents. It requires the adoption of a set of attitudes and behaviors by people to reduce risk to all activities involving domestic, captive/exotic and wild animals and their products". Moreover bio-security can also slow down the transmission of endemic pathogens (yeasts, bacteria, parasites and fungi) thus limiting the spread of diseases in a herd / flock, region / country. Good herd/ flock bio-security is therefore essential to protect the herd/ flock.

In its common usage, bio-security refers to the protection of health through avoidance of disease. Bio-security is defined as: "The implementation of measures that reduce the risk of the introduction and spread of disease agents; it requires the adoption of a set of attitudes and behaviors by people to reduce risk in all activities involving domestic, captive/exotic and wild animals and their products" Hence, bio-security is presented under two components: bio-exclusion (or external bio-security) combines all activities to preclude the introduction of disease to the farm; and bio-containment (or internal bio-security) refers to efforts to prevent the spread of a disease within the farm herd and to other farms.

In a world where people, animals and goods relevant to domestic animals (DAs) move globally, the risk of disease spread is increasing. Global markets have brought increased international trade and economic opportunities, making international information and standards on bio-security essential. OIE defines international standards that are recognized by the World Trade Organization (WTO) under the agreement on the application of sanitary and phyto-sanitary (SPS) measures and that aim to enable international trade without compromising animal health. FAO's mandate is to raise levels of nutrition, improve agricultural productivity, improve the lives of rural populations and contribute to growth of the world economy. Bio-security is a tool that contributes to achieving these objectives.

9.2 Key elements of bio-security

The following are the three main elements of bio-security:

9.2.1 Segregation

Segregation is the first and most important element of bio-security. It involves keeping potentially infected animals and materials away from uninfected animals. Segregation is regarded as the most effective step in achieving the required levels of bio-security. If a pathogen does not enter a holding, no infection can take place. No animals or materials should enter or leave a pig holding unless absolutely necessary: this includes not only pigs, but also other species od DAs (including humans) that may be infected with pathogens and that can also infect pigs. Segregation involves the creation of barriers and the control of what passes through them. This includes such measures as enforcing the changing of footwear and clothing for all people crossing the barrier, and restricting the entry of vehicles. Segregation is the basis of most bio-security measures, from the farm-gate to individual pig sheds. Segregation measures include controlling the entry of pigs from outside farms, markets or villages; implementing quarantine for newly purchased animals; limiting the number of sources of replacement stocks; fencing a farm area and controlling access for people, as well as birds, bats, rodents, cats and dogs; maintaining adequate distances between farms; providing footwear and clothing to be worn only on the farm; and using an all-in-all-out management system.

9.2.2 Cleaning

The next most effective step in bio-security is cleaning of the whole farm and not only pig houses/ sties. Most pathogen contamination on physical objects is contained in fecal material, urine or secretions that adhere to the surface; cleaning will therefore remove most of the contaminating pathogen. Any materials that must pass through the segregation barrier (in either direction) should be thoroughly cleaned. This means that there should be no visible dirt on the surface of materials. Soap, water and a brush are adequate for small objects, but a high-pressure washer (of 110 to 130 bar) is needed for large vehicles, such as trucks or tractors. The difficulty of properly cleaning such large complex items emphasizes the need for segregation as the first and most effective method of protection.

9.2.3 Disinfection

The final step of bio-security is disinfection. The disinfection is the application after thorough cleansing procedures intended to destroy the infectious or parasitic agents related to animal diseases including zoonoses. This applies to premises, vehicles and different objects which may have been directly or indirectly contaminated. Disinfection is important when performed consistently and correctly, but should be regarded as a final "polishing" step in bio-security, used after effective and comprehensive cleaning.

Before purchasing new reproductive females and males even piglets of either sex, their medical history should be gathered and a veterinary consultation should be obtained on the seller's farm. Before purchase, it is important to test a representative sample of the pigs with serological or molecular techniques to detect the percentage/ level of sub-clinical disease, and to place animals in acclimatization quarantine to identify any incubating diseases. The unit's bio-security protocols are sufficient to prevent disease entry and identify an outbreak as quickly as possible: Molecular diagnostic techniques that are now available can be used on boar studs. There are examples of PRRS virus infection being detected in boar studs before semen transmission to downstream herds occurs.

The physical location of the herds should be planned to maintain sufficient distances from neighboring farms and frequently used roads: As with small-scale confined pig production, the buffer distance varies according to the size of the farm.

For aerosol transmission, the same rule applies as for the previous system: For units where significant investment in domestic animals (DAs) health has occurred, incoming air is sometimes filtered in an attempt to reduce the risk of airborne infection. Visitor control needs a major focus, as both can bring pathogens to the farm. Only essential people who work in the sheds/ sties have access to the farm and animals, and they follow the guidelines that recommend changing of clothing and footwear, and hand-washing or showering.

Decontamination of vehicles is necessary before their entry to the farm and drive-ways. Parking areas should be designed to prevent cross-contamination of workers and farm vehicles. Vehicle that transport pigs among farms are a major source of disease risk, so protocols for the effective disinfection of trailers and trucks are necessary.

One of the most common route of transmission for infectious agents is direct pig-to-pig contact: movement of infected pigs in close physical contact with non-infected pigs is decisive in transmitting diseases. Disease transmission through infected semen is well-documented. The role of people in disease transmission has been studied closely over the last decade: they can transport pathogens on footwear, clothing, hands, etc. People can carry viruses on their nasal mucosae (nasal carriers) without being infected. They can also be infected and shed pathogens as healthy or sick carriers.

Animal diseases that are known to spread primarily through human activities can be prevented and controlled through the application of bio-security measures along the production and marketing chain, together with increased awareness and education. It is this notion that makes bio-security so critically important in the prevention, control and elimination of trans-boundary animal diseases (TADs), with the focus on changing the habits and behaviors of people in such a way that the risk of disease transmission is decreased. A key aspect is to work with people to adopt bio-security measures and to develop with them sets of safe practices in production that are seen as practical, cost-effective and sustainable. Vehicles and equipment can be instrumental in spreading diseases. Airborne transmission is more difficult to document, but has been studied experimentally. As some pathogens can survive in meat waste, specific attention must be paid to the use of food wastes in feeding pigs. Feed, water and bedding can all become contaminated and play a role in maintaining diseases. Faces from infected pigs can contain large quantities of pathogenic viruses, bacteria or parasites: thus the application of manure to agricultural land may introduce pathogens into the human food chain and ecosystem, if due care is not taken during storage and spreading. Birds, rodents, stray dogs and cats, wildlife and feral pigs, together with arthropods, can all be potential carriers, whether through mechanical transmission or by being infected.

9.3 Designing a bio-security plan for a pig farm

Bio-security is extremely important to ensure proper health and production, in a pig farm. There are two levels of bio-security viz. at the International/ national level and at the farm level. The farm level bio-security would depend on the location of the farm. Ideally a pig production unit should be located in an isolated area away from other pig or even other domestic animals (DAs) farms. However, this may not be always possible and measures to control movement of man and material and ensuring that at the entrance disinfection measures are available. It would be preferable if all the persons entering the farm take a shower and change their cloths to those only used at the farm. The shoes should also be changed or at least cover with a disposable plastic cover. Sufficient space more than the covered area and loafing area may be provided at the farm which may be vegetated with trees and shrubs. The shed should be cleaned regularly preferably with disinfectant.

The herd size should be according to the housing space available and single sty should carry preferably a smaller herd not exceeding 20 and sufficient feeding and watering space should be provided to avoid competition. The leftover feed should be regularly removed and disposed off and feeding troughs should be thoroughly cleaned with disinfectant.

The new pigs should be introduced only after proper quarantine for a period of four weeks and during this period they should be vaccinated against the prevailing diseases and treated against internal and external parasites.

In most farms the pig catchers have to enter the farm for catching the pigs for marketing. Since they may have also gone to some other farm, they should preferably go through a disinfection and change of clothes before entering the farm. The visitors to the farm should, as far as possible, be avoided and if necessary should be made to walk through the corridor and be avoided their entry in the pig sties. They should also be made to clean and disinfect and wear protective cloths.

The farm should be properly fenced to avoid entry of domestic and wild animals. All animals showing any abnormal behavior, diarrhea or high temperature should be segregated, properly examined by veterinarian and treated. All dead animals should be removed immediately and disposed of by burning or deep burial with lime under and above the carcass. The sty should be thoroughly disinfected and other animals in the sty may be removed to another sty for some time.

The key strategic objectives of a farm bio-security plan

The key strategic objectives of a farm bio-security plan are to:

i) Prevent the introduction of infectious disease agents to pigs.

ii) Reduce the spread of an infectious disease among pigs on premises already contaminated with a disease agent.

iii) Prevent the escape and spread of disease agents already present on pig premises to other un-infected DA populations

iv) Minimize the incidence and spread of microorganisms of public health significance.

Bio-security is about managing risk to meet the objectives stated above. It is important that an assessment be conducted for each enterprise to establish what level of risk exists in each phase of its operations, and to identify and implement appropriate control measures to these risks. Bio-security is an integral and proactive part of any successful pig production system. Bio-security can have a preventative impact, which can enable producers to protect their assets. Bio-security refers to those measures taken to prevent or control the introduction and spread of infectious agents to a herd. Such infectious agents, whether they cause clinical or subclinical disease, significantly reduce the productivity, profitability and long term financial viability of a pig operation. These procedures cover areas of risk common to most pig farms, intensive / extensive, large / small herds, and appropriate measures to minimize these risks. When undertaking the risk assessment to determine farm-specific bio-security measures, it is important to take into account all factors that may impact on the bio-security of the production area. These factors include:

i) Location and layout of farm and production area
ii) Source of feed and water supply
iii) Disease status of the region in which the pig farm is located
iv) Proximity to other production areas with pigs or other DAs
v) Presence and type of wildlife
vi) Customer/supplier interactions and customer requirements (customer/ supplier interactions include pick-ups and deliveries of DAs and feed, as well as interactions with service/ trades personnel, industry personnel and contractors). Customer requirements may also affect the biosecurity measures needed.

Routs of disease spread in pigs

Live animals

i) Transfer of pigs from one production area to another
ii) Dead pig disposal or waste materials from farm having an outbreak of an infectious disease

Semen

i) Semen from boar stations
ii) Within herd transmission of venereal transmitted diseases when using on-farm artificial insemination (AI) with own boars
iii) Semen imported from other regions within the country or abroad.

Other animals

i) Wild birds

ii) Feral and DAs, other DAs, predators and pets

iii) Insects

iv) Rodents

v) Domestic or wild birds

People

i) Farm personnel and family members living on site

ii) Contractors, maintenance personnel, neighbors, service personnel and visitors

iii) Dirt/manure/contaminants carried on hands, boots, clothing, dirty hair, vehicles and equipment

iv) Dirt/manure/contaminants carried on cars, trucks, tractors, scales, husbandry equipment

Air

i) Transmission as an aerosol or dust, feed and water

ii) Contamination with faeces/urine from contact with avian or other DA species

iii) Raw materials

iv) Post production contamination or spoilage during transport and storage

v) Kitchen waste or other food scraps should not be fed to pigs. This is 'prohibited feed' and is also known as swill.

Level 1 – Routine bio-security procedures

1. Movements of pigs and other animals

i) Drivers and other transport personnel must not enter pig farm or free range areas or designated 'clean areas' unless they have complied with the on-farm bio-security arrangements.

ii) Vehicles are not allowed into 'clean' areas unless authorized.

iii) Before commencing movement in and out of farm, drivers must complete the transporter's declaration on the valid movement document accompanying the consignment. Drivers must provide a copy of the movement document with the signed transporter's declaration to the producer.

iv) Pigs must be identified prior to transport.

v) All introduced DAs must be inspected for signs of disease on arrival.

vi) All introduced breeding stock male/ female piglets or boars/ sows with an unknown health status must be isolated from other pigs and observed for signs of disease for a minimum of 21 days.

vii) All pigs exhibited at shows must be isolated / disinfected and observed for signs of disease for a minimum of 21 days after returning to the farm of origin.

viii) Load-outs of pigs should be at the farm perimeter wherever possible. Where this is not possible, the race and loading facility should be designed to minimize the possibility of pigs running off the truck and back into the shed.

ix) Semen deliveries should only come from a reliable verified source such as accredited farms.

x) Trucks should be cleaned, disinfected and left to dry between consignments when moving pigs from a farm not owned by the same entity. Cleaning should be done after each day of use when transporting pigs as a minimum requirement.

xi) If cattle, sheep or goats are brought in to graze around the pig sheds or into the outdoor range areas, this should be done only for as limited time as necessary and with the awareness that it may pose a potential risk of disease transfer. Such stock should be retained on the property for a minimum period of two weeks after grazing within close proximity of pigs in order to allow any signs of infectious disease to be seen before they are transferred off the farm.

xii) Cats should be kept out of the production area as far as is practically possible.

xiii) Commercial poultry operations should not be present on the same property, or if they are should be completely separated from the pig operation with an adequate buffer zone.

xiv) Dead pigs must be disposed of according to regulatory requirements and good bio-security practices.

2. People, equipment and vehicle movements

To minimize the risk of introduction of disease or contaminants by production personnel, equipments and vehicle movements, the recommended practices are:

i) Hands even of the farm workers should be cleaned before entering the production site and on leaving the production site.

ii) Production area personnel should wear laundered clean clothes each day at the commencement of their work.

iii) Shoes and outer shoe cover that are worn in the production area should not be worn or taken outside this area as they are the most likely method for disease spread by personnel.

iv) Staff should always work from 'least risk production areas i.e. from 'cleaner' production areas with higher bio-security standards (e.g. youngest, most vulnerable pigs or healthy production area) to 'high risk' production areas, i.e. those with lower bio-security standards. In an emergency, access may be made from high risk production areas with lower standards of bio-security after a shower and complete change of clothing.

v) All contractors, suppliers, service personnel and visitors must agree to comply with the entry conditions for visitors.

vi) Contractors who have had contact with pigs that day, who are required to enter sheds populated with pigs to undertake emergency repair and/or maintenance, must shower thoroughly and change clothing and boots.

vii) Hand washing facilities should be available at all production area entrances and must be used before entering.

viii) If visitors wear their own boots into the sheds or any designated 'clean' area, the soles of the boots should be scraped clear of any organic matter before cleaning and disinfecting. Alternatively, shed boots or disposable plastic covers must be provided.

ix) All equipment should be visibly clean and, where practical, the exterior treated by wet disinfection or water and detergent or other disinfectant after use and, where possible, between animals.

x) All visitors should park their vehicles outside the production area, unless it is essential the vehicle be taken on site.

xi) Trucks carting new or old bedding materials, feed and other supplies should be cleaned and disinfected wherever possible between visits to different production areas.

3. Water, feed and bedding

3.1 Water

To ensure that water used in pig sheds for drinking, cooling and cleaning, is of a standard suitable for DAs and should not introduce pathogens to the pigs. The use of a suitable water supply is important for good bio-security. If water treatment is required, water with a high level of organic matter is unsuitable for chlorination alone. Ultraviolet treatment is also of little use for turbid water. It may be necessary to seek expert advice to ensure a safe water supply. Any water treatment process should be monitored regularly.

i) Drinking water quality should be maintained at a suitable standard for pigs.

ii) All surface water should be tested and if necessary treated before being used as drinking water for pigs.

iii) Expert advice should be sought on water treatment options if water testing shows the available water to be of unsuitable quality.

iv) A treated water supply should be kept in a closed system from the point of treatment to the drinker.

3.2 Feed and bedding

To manage the introduction and movement of pig feed stuffs and bedding in a way that minimizes the risk of introducing or spreading infectious diseases, the following standards and recommended practices may be followed:

i) Prohibit pig feed or any food scraps that contain meat, other matter from animals, or any other substance prohibited under state and territory legislation must not be fed to pigs.

ii) All feed and bedding provided for pigs should be accompanied by a commodity vendor declaration stating that it is free from contaminants and fit for the purpose.

iii) Feed spills should be cleaned up as soon as practicable. Feed attracts birds and rodents to the production area.

iv) Pig feed should be stored in a manner that prevents contamination by DAs, vermin, insects, wildlife, feral and other animals.

v) Pig feed should be inspected on delivery for evidence of any pests and contaminants and should not be accepted.

4. Pest and vermin control

To minimize the potential for introduction of infectious agents and pathogens by feral animals and pests, in particular rodents, through their presence in the production area, bait stations or traps for rodents, cats, flies and other insects should be set as required and meet regulatory requirements for use where appropriate.

5. Management

5.1 Training

To ensure awareness to employees, training in all relevant bio-security requirements, the following standards may be followed:

i) A controlled entrance to the pig farm through which visitors, animals and transport movements are admitted,

ii) A record of all visitors, animals introduced and transport vehicle movements,

iii) Hand washing and/or shower facilities and/or boots and clothing provided to all authorized visitors prior to entering the piggery,

iv) An employee Bio-security Declaration signed by all staff confirming their adherence to the farm bio-security procedures,

v) Ensure all equipment used around pigs or brought into pig housing is cleaned and, where practical, disinfected.

vi) The bio-security plan must, wherever possible, also include the designation of 'clean' and 'dirty' areas,

vii) Warning signs displayed on entry gates and/or shed doors, along with locked entrances where appropriate, to discourage unauthorized entry of pigs brought from outside and feed truck drivers or unauthorized visitors.

viii) Must have a documented herd health plan to manage the risk of infectious diseases entering the piggery and to treat existing disease problems promptly and efficiently.

5.2 Record keeping

To assist early detection of animal health issues and the response to any bio-security breach, the recommended practices are:

i) A register should be maintained recording training of farm personnel in bio-security requirements.

ii) All pig mortalities and cases of disease must be recorded to assist monitoring for any unusual animal health problems potentially indicating a bio-security breach.

5.3 Herd health requirements

To assist management of disease risk on farm, the following standards may be maintained:

i) Inspect all pigs at least once daily for any signs of ill health

ii) Separate sick pigs into sick pens where possible and treat appropriately

6. Required protection for ensuring biosecurity

To design and maintain pig production areas, including sheds, that will assist in providing a biosecure area the following practices are recommended:

- A sketch, map, plan or photo of the layout of the farm, showing the production area, sheds, paddocks, access roads and gates should be created and maintained up-to-date. 'Clean' areas to which restricted access applies and 'dirty' areas should be clearly shown. The feed silos and loading area are generally considered 'dirty' areas and parts of the production site where pigs are housed is designated as 'clean' areas.
- The main entrance to the production area should be capable of being closed off to vehicle traffic and should display appropriate signages including 'Bio-secure Area' No Entry Unless Authorized' or similar wording. In addition, signage must direct visitors to contact the producer before proceeding, i.e. telephone number and/or enquire at house/office.
- There should be a parking area for vehicles not entering the production area.
- There should be a changeover area away, and separate from the production area, with clean protective clothing and boots provided by the farm.
- All pig housing, bedding and feed sheds should be designed and maintained so as to limit access of vermin and entry of wild birds, feral animals and other pests as far as practical.
- Trees and shrubs should be slightly away from the immediate shed area to deter wildlife. Vegetation should be carefully selected to minimize wild bird attraction.

7. Customer or farm specific additional bio-security requirements

To build on the generic pork production, bio-security requirements which reflect specific additional requirements and operational procedures, should be added to the farm bio-security plan.

Level 2 – High risk bio-security procedures

To protect the pig farm from the increased threat of pathogens being introduced from the outside during a suspected outbreak of an emergency or serious endemic disease, the following measures should be taken:

1. Action plan for suspected emergency animal disease

Each pig farmer should establish and document clear guidelines regarding the circumstances when an emergency animal disease occurs on the farm, alert should be raised, movement of pigs must cease immediately.

2. Facilities

i) Gates of the farm must be kept locked where ever possible or shall have proper foot bath facilities.

ii) Facilities for the cleaning and disinfection of equipment coming on and off the production area must be in place.

3. Personnel

i) No non-essential visitors to enter the production areas.

ii) Repairs and maintenance - no routine work, only emergency work to be carried out.

4. Operational

i) Any vehicle which must enter the farm must be washed and disinfected at the farm entrance before and after going into the farm (e.g. feed trucks). Vehicle driver cabins must also be sanitized inside (e.g. a household spray type disinfectant).

ii) No pigs, litter or manure to be moved on or off properties until the disease status is clarified by a veterinarian.

iii) A complete change of clothes, footwear, hair covering and breathing protection is required. Used protective clothing and all used personal protection equipment must remain on the farm and disposed of in case of plastic gloves/ shoe covers and other clothes wore in the shed be thoroughly washed.

5. Standard operating procedures (SOPs) for disease emergencies

- Visitors must first report to the piggery office and complete the visitors' log book
- Visitors must wear protective clothing and boots provided by the farm
- Visitors must clean/sanitize hands before entering sheds and preferably wear disposable plastic gloves.

Carcass Management

From an environmental perspective, rendering and composting are the preferred methods for carcass disposal (dead pig disposal, including disposal of stillborn piglets and afterbirth). Suitable alternatives may include incineration and burial. Irrespective of the method chosen, dead pigs should be immediately removed from the pig house so the carcass is not accessed by other pigs and disposed of within 24 hours of death. Poor carcass management practices may contaminate groundwater and surface water, cause bad odor, spread infectious diseases. Well-managed carcass composting is an environmentally acceptable method and has the advantage of producing a soil amendment. Large carcasses need slitting before placing them in the compost pile to reduce the gasses that cause bloating, thus preventing bloated carcasses rising out of the pit. When a carcass bay is full, a new one should be started. The carcasses in the full bay are then allowed to decompose for around three months. When the compost is used as a fertilizer, it should be spread evenly onto land at environmentally sustainable rates. To minimize the risk of grazing DAs contracting salmonellosis or mastitis, they should be excluded from these areas for at least three weeks after the compost is spread.

Rendering

Rendering is an excellent carcasses management method because there is little risk of adverse environmental impacts. Rendered carcasses can also provide saleable meat and bone meal. However, this method is only economically viable if there is a nearby rendering plant willing to receive the carcasses from other pig farms. This however has been banned in India and such a feed cannot be used for feeding DAs.

Burial

Burial is a common method of disposing carcasses. However, it should only be used where rendering or composting is not feasible. Burial is not the preferred method because:

i) The carcasses decompose slowly and need covering with lime and soil to avoid odour problems and scavenging by feral animals.

ii) Burial pits fill quickly and continually need replacement.

iii) Nutrients and bacteria can leach into and contaminate groundwater, particularly if there is shallow groundwater and inappropriate sealing of the bottom of the pits.

iv) Storm water run-off from pits can contaminate surface water and land can become contaminated. This should be properly sealed with earth.

To avoid these problems:

i) Large carcasses should be split to minimize bloating.

ii) The pit bases should be at least 2 m above the water table at all times.

iii) Pits should be situated on low permeability soils and / or low risk sites.

iv) Carcasses need to be well covered with soil, or other suitable material, each day to avoid scavenging by feral animals and to prevent odor and further clay should be compacted over filled pits

Burning or Incineration

While biologically the safest carcass management method, incineration is generally not ideal because:

i) It needs to be performed efficiently and effectively to ensure that it is complete.

ii) Needs to avoid complaints about smoke odor and particulates.

iii) It is not energy efficient and generates greenhouse gases.

iv) It is expensive.

Mass Carcass Disposal

However, all pig keepers should identify a disposal site and have a contingency plan for managing the high death rates that may occur as part of an infectious disease outbreak. State government veterinary officers have the main responsibility and resources to combat an infectious disease incursion or endemic disease outbreak. They should be contacted immediately if a disease outbreak is suspected. The relevant state government department should be consulted regarding selection of a disposal method and site.

If mass carcass disposal is needed, burial is often the preferred method as it is quick, cheap, relatively easily organized and, if properly done, environmentally clean. If burial is to be used, a suitable site may be located. It should be readily accessible, be well separated from sensitive areas and be of a soil type that does not drain readily. The pits should be as deep as possible while ensuring that the base is at least 2 m above the water table.

Development of a practical bio-security plan to a pig farm

The bio-security measures would vary from one pig farm to another depending upon the functions, whether it is a nucleus farm maintaining purebreds for multiplication or is undertaking selection for genetic improvement. The next levels are multipliers farm which purchases the breeding stock from the nucleus and produces boars and guilt for sale. There may be boars for providing service or collection or processing of semen for AI. The multiplier farm may sell young piglets at weaning to be raised by finishing farm.

A veterinarian providing house services should require about the effectiveness of the health measures, any recent disease incidence, proper survival and growth and any abnormal behaviors of the pigs. Based on the history and his own observations and the health cover being provided, he should advice any modification in the health cover, if required.

"Prevention is always better than cure" and preventive measures are cheaper than the treatment. Since pigs are highly prolific and fast growing, would suffer more often both from infectious and non-infectious diseases. Proper surveillance and monitoring of diseases in a herd would help in their timely control and eradication and save from mortality and morbidity and extra expenditure on providing treatment to animals.

i) ***Pig production systems***: The implementation of bio-security measures in scavenging pig production systems is constrained by the producers' limited capacity to invest resources and time, and by the nature of scavenging pig production where it is exposed to all kind of infectious materials. However, there are simple measures that can be recommended and that are mainly related to segregation: new pigs introduced into a location must be free from disease, and particular attention is required when they are purchased from a market. The use of quarantine is very important. There is also concern over sows and boars that are moved from one location to another for mating. The health status of the boars needs to be known, particularly regarding diseases of concern. It is common practice for poor pig farmers to sell animals for slaughter as soon as disease is suspected. The marketing of sick animals is a serious disease risk to human beings, as these incubating or excreting sick pigs disseminate diseases, particularly when they are sold at live-animal markets. This practice should be prevented. The use of untreated pig swill must be avoided, and is often prohibited by national regulations. In the case of unusual pig deaths, veterinary services should be informed, so that immediate actions can be taken to control the disease outbreaks. Proper disposal of carcasses by burying, composting or burning is also crucial. Cleaning of night shelters and equipment must be emphasized.

ii) ***Small-scale confined pig production system:*** In small-scale confined pig production system, measures will focus on the three elements of biosecurity. An important difference between small-scale confined and scavenging pig production is that confinement facilitates allow segregation. The measures proposed for scavenging pigs are also valid for small-scale confined pig production. Newly purchased pigs should be kept for a minimum of 30 days in a quarantine pen.

   In this system, additional measures can be introduced. The premises of the pig farm can be controlled. An all-in-all-out management system could be used. Proper fencing and measures to control contact with birds, rodents, cats and dogs can be promoted. It is important to develop protocols for the farm, to which visitors must strictly adhere to. With confined pigs, it is possible to control access for vehicles and people, including drivers and feed providers. Authorized visitors, particularly those dealing with pigs - including other farmers - should be provided with specific clothing and clean footwear by the farm being visited, and should wash their hands on entry. All instruments or equipment that is likely to come into contact with pigs should be assigned to the farm and kept clean.

The importance of regular and thorough cleaning of the pig unit is often not fully understood. Manure should be removed from the pens every day, unless there are slatted floors or an equivalent. Contact with manure, urine and straw bedding from sick and dead animals should be avoided. After cleaning, the use of disinfectant should be promoted. When a batch of same-aged pigs leaves a building, the room should be thoroughly cleaned and disinfected. Vehicles, especially those used to transport pigs, should be thoroughly cleaned and disinfected before returning to or visiting other farms. A safe pig loading bay will limit movement of vehicles on the farm.

iii) ***Large-scale confined and intensive production systems***: In large-scale confined and intensive production systems, the same principles apply as for the previously discussed, but the impact of disease has the potential to be proportionally higher. The physical location of herds should be planned to maintain adequate distances from neighboring farms and frequently used roads. For aerosol transmission, the same rules applies as for the previous system. For units where significant investment in DAs health has occurred, filtration of incoming air is sometimes employed in an attempt to reduce the risk of airborne infection. Standards should be developed for the purchase of incoming live animals. When practicing AI, the health status of the AI unit should match that of the recipient herd, and its bio-security protocols should be adequate. The control of visitors is a major focus, who can bring pathogens to the farm. Training and updating of staff by veterinarians and technicians specialized in disease control is necessary. A number of disease control measures and techniques are now available to control relevant pathogens in commercial farms. The biggest challenge is often to ensure proper implementation of good husbandry practices. Progressive eradication of pathogens contributes to regional bio-security by lowering the regional disease risk. Followed to its logical conclusion, this process can result in eradication of disease from the region or country.

Bio-security for large-scale outdoor production systems needs to focus on the control of feedstuffs, water and pasture contamination, wildlife and human visitors. Other factors such as transportation and sources of breeding stock also need to be considered, as the risks are the same as in the other production systems.

Intermediaries, service providers and transporters are the key links along pig production and marketing chains. Their potential roles in disease transmission-but also as champions for bio-security-is important; they must therefore be fully involved in the implementation of bio-security programmes.

Slaughterhouses are another important element in the marketing chain where all three elements of bio-security must be implemented, with a major focus on bio-containment.

To maintain a high health status at AI centers, it is essential that the boars purchased are of verified disease-free status. The implementation of a quality assurance scheme in these enterprises should be a priority.

Live-animal markets are obvious mixing points and a potential source of disease spread: bio-containment is crucial at these sites, and contact among animals from different farms must be controlled. To limit the risk of disease spread, animals that have not been sold should not be reintroduced back into the home herd without a quarantine period. Wastewater and slurries need to be managed properly. However, such markets are also a useful location for disseminating and collecting information.

9.4 Bio-security Measures for Service Providers and Along Marketing Chains

Artificial insemination centers and boar keepers

The main concerns arise when the health status of boars at AI centers and on boar farms is not controlled, and when hygiene of semen collection is neglected. One boar may produce from 20 to more than 50 semen doses per week, so introduction of pathogens through this pathway is of a major significance. The number of semen doses produced and the area in which they are distributed make AI centers a major potential source of infection. Practices such as pooling semen from multiple boars exacerbate the health risks to recipient farms. In cases of natural mating provided by an external boar, animal movements are necessary, for example, sows in heat are moved to the boar farm (or vice versa). Such movements between farms create significant health risks, and animal quarantine before reintroduction into the herd is usually not feasible. Maximum efforts must constantly be directed to maintaining a high health status at AI centers through the purchase of boars whose disease-free health status has been verified. The implementation of quality assurance in these enterprises should be a priority. AI centers should be officially controlled, and veterinary services' certification against transmissible diseases (Pseudorabies, CSF, ASF, etc.) may be required. Veterinary authorities should plan regular audits of AI facilities and practices. Traceability and quality control of the semen doses must be in place. Promoting and facilitating farmers' investments in boar studs and training in pig AI may be a viable solution in developing and transition countries. Locally, there would be a bio-security benefit from the decreased circulation of live animals from farm to farm.

Brokers and transporters

Service providers may understand the risk of disease spread, but may be under pressure to visit multiple farms on a single day, or may take short-cuts on decontamination. Intermediaries and collectors link the different segments and systems in the pig sector. They are potential transmitters and must implement appropriate bio-security measures at all times. Brokers and transporters should not carry animals that are showing obvious signs of illness or that come from a farm known to be affected by a disease, unless they follow instructions from the veterinary services and appropriate measures are taken before and after transportation.

Vehicles may transmit pathogens when manure containing disease agents is attached to inside the body or tyres. Pig industry service providers should not have to enter pig buildings; if they do so, they must wear specific protective clothing and footwear and follow all visitor protocols. All clothing and footwear must be cleaned and disinfected or be disposable. Commercial incentives must not override bio-security, and practices such as having visitors document their previous farm visits help to ensure compliance with bio-security protocols.

Slaughterhouses

Hygiene and bio-security standards vary widely in slaughtering facilities. In addition, many pigs are slaughtered on-farm, for local consumption and with no meat inspection. Slaughterhouse workers, butchers providing services to individuals, and producers who slaughter their own pigs are all at risk of contracting zoonotic diseases. On premises where pigs are slaughtered, visitors' access and the entry of animals other than those slaughtered must be controlled. By-products from slaughterhouses, such as blood and offal, are sometimes used to feed pigs in the vicinity, thereby creating significant risk of disease transfer. Public investment in environmental protection, urban sanitation, water supply and drainage or hygiene in slaughterhouses is often inadequate, thus increasing the risk of disease transmission. Slaughterhouses are a risk point for the spread of animal zoonotic diseases. Animals from different species and of different origin are all concentrated in one location and there is important movement of people and vehicles. All incoming animals must be carefully observed for any signs of disease; many notifiable diseases are first detected at the time of slaughter. Animals with clinical signs of disease, such as a fever, should not enter the food chain. Slaughterhouse management involves the enforcement of measures for strict hygiene and bio-security, including:

i) cleaning and disinfecting the entire slaughterhouse premises at the end of each working day to ensure that it is free of manure, hair and other debris that may harbor pathogens;
ii) thorough cleaning and disinfection of all vehicles used for transporting live pigs, and of the wheels and undercarriages of all other vehicles before they leave the premises;
iii) banning visits to pig farms by operators and their staff;
iv) installing a pest management programme;
v) monitoring the health status of all workers.

Application of these basic measures is feasible in all pig production, slaughter and marketing systems.

Live-animal markets and exhibitions

Live-animal markets, particularly those in developing countries, are essential venues for trade. The animals sold are mainly piglets or young replacement breeding stock, such as gilts. Live-animal markets are clear mixing points of animals from different sources and a potential source of disease spread. Moreover, as traders are often intermediaries/ collectors who collect animals from different locations, pig producers do not have any assurance about the health and sanitary status of the animals. Bio-containment of infection is vital at these sites, and contacts among animals of different origins must be controlled. As far as possible, animals that have been taken to the market but not sold should not be reintroduced into the home herd without proper quarantine period. Waste water and slurries must also be managed correctly. Live-animal markets could play a positive role in the control of pig diseases as places where information can be disseminated and collected. Active surveillance for diseases can also be carried out at the market place, but its efficiency depends on having a traceability system with farm or pig identification. Exhibitions where high-value animals are shown to the public are also key risk points for animal disease transmission; particular attention must be paid to observing an appropriate quarantine period for the exhibited animals before they re-enter the home herd.

9.5 Challenges in the implementation of bio-security measures

Farmers' ability to implement on-farm bio-security measures depends on the characteristics of the production system they operate, their knowledge of technical matters and the availability of resources. Controlling diseases in pig farms is a continuous process, which requires investments. The introduction of new bio-security measures to a farm may also require important changes in husbandry practices. Global bio-security issues are relevant to all environments, but may be particularly challenging in developing and transition countries.

Social and economic factors

The pig production systems in a given area are largely determined by the demands that people and society place on them. Knowledge of the diversity of systems and understanding of the people involved in pig production and their motivations for keeping animals will help the development of strategies for implementing sustainable bio-security measures on-farm and along production and marketing chain. Important issues for producers and other stakeholders involved in pig production are their asset bases, their perceptions of risk, their interactions with the wider community (including their own roles and responsibilities within the community, and with the government), and prevalent consumer demands. Tools such as livelihood analysis, value chain mapping and cost/benefit or cost-effectiveness analysis are helpful to understand these issues. Farmers' motivations and the degree to which pigs contribute to his income portfolios are identified through livelihood analyses; this increases understanding of the resources available and the drivers for or against investment in bio-security measures. Value chain mapping and institutional analyses provide insight into the people involved in pig production, and therefore into who should be involved in developing bio-security measures. When designing and implementing measures at the household level, it is important to undertake a financial evaluation using, for instance, cost-effectiveness or cost : benefit analysis. Cost-effectiveness enables the stakeholder to define the acceptable level of risk and then look for the most economical method of achieving this. This means considering the set-up and recurrent costs for the proposed bio-security interventions, and the costs of disrupting the production system. When designing interventions, their socio-cultural and religious acceptability should be considered, as should the new measures' impacts on the roles and responsibilities of men and women. Cost/benefit analysis also requires an estimate of the potential benefits to the producer, such as increased production, increased efficiency or decreased risk of loss on investment. This process requires producers to have reasonably accurate records of costs and income over a sufficient period. Understanding the impacts of disease on society and communicating these effectively throughout the production and marketing chains will be essential for improving the uptake of bio-security measures.

Sharing of responsibilities between the private and public sectors

The maintenance of good health in DAs through appropriate bio-security measures is important to both the private and public sectors: all the private stakeholders involved in the production and marketing chain, the ministries of health and agriculture, and national/ regional trade organizations. When recommending the implementation of bio-security measures, it is necessary to consider which sector should pay for what and to determine the appropriate balance between incentives for voluntary implementation and regulations. In recent years, a debate on whether to classify animal health as a public or a private good has emerged. There is now consensus that prevention and control of major diseases, particularly those that are trans-boundary and innovative in nature, should be totally or partially considered as a public good. For optimal implementation of bio-security measures, the private and public sectors need to collaborate closely and with mutual trust. Prevention and control programmes should be supported by public funds or by a combination of public and private funds. The public sector has a strong motive for decreasing the risk of disease introduction and spread, because of the imperative to limit impacts on the national economy. Private animal producers have an equally strong motive for decreasing risk, as they bear the brunt of the impacts through mortality and morbidity of their stock. Producers also face recurrent losses due to endemic diseases, and this may be the strongest reason for them to apply bio-security measures.

Animal health systems and veterinary services

Developed countries have progressively improved the health status of their national herds through advances in Veterinary Science and the establishment of appropriate animal health systems comprising public and private veterinary infrastructure and services to the livestock sector. Some of the important diseases DAs have been eradicated at the national level; measures to safeguard against their reintroduction have been initiated. Other endemic diseases are under surveillance or targeted for eradication, where possible. Farmers have access to both public and private veterinary services, while research institutions and public and private extension services foster continuous improvements in livestock industries. The situation in developing countries varies. The DA sector is characterized by a large number of small producers, for whom DA rearing is sole a major source of livelihood. There is an absence of influential livestock owners' associations and there is often a need to enhance the capacity and resources of public veterinary services so as to improve the quality and coverage of services provided to DA keepers. The importance of subsistence DA production, market failures, the dynamics of contagious diseases, economic constraints and institutional weaknesses all need to be considered and understood when programmes to improve animal health systems are designed.

Education and extension services

The availability of an appropriately trained and skilled workforce is a critical requirement in developing a DA sector, and research, education and extension must be undertaken for all stakeholders, after their needs have been identified. In many regions, animal farming is considered a speculative side-activity, especially in urban and peri-urban areas. Adapting and disseminating training and extension material is still a challenge for national extension services, but they can be assisted by universities, national research centers, non-governmental organizations (NGOs) or international organizations.

The role and importance of communication in promoting bio-security

Communication is the process of mediating dialogue among all relevant stakeholders, to identify the attitudes, perceptions and needs of each participant. It involves formulating explanations, recommendations and messages about the policies and activities that best address the collective interest. Communication is also a tool for advocacy, promoting the importance of bio-security for DA and livelihoods in key sectors, especially among policy-makers and in DA farming communities. Communication is essential for the "buy-in" of all parties to bio-security policies and activities, and for ensuring that these are subsequently adopted and implemented effectively. Communication is also a way of creating an environment or culture that supports activities designed to satisfy the collective interest. Communication interventions for bio-security in pig production need to bring together the various stakeholders – including pig keepers, handlers, technical specialists and policy-makers - to facilitate the sharing of information and opinions on an equal footing among them. It should aim to ensure that policies are not imposed in a top-down fashion, and that those who will be affected by and expected to implement the policies in question have their concerns and needs taken into consideration. Given the wide range of pig production and marketing systems, and the rapidly expanding and transnational trade in pork products, the core areas that need to be supported by communication, advocacy and social mobilization interventions include:

i) promoting and establishing bio-security as professional and social rules along the entire production/marketing/consumption chain;

ii) promoting community-based surveillance and monitoring of disease by producers and service providers, and facilitating active public engagement in control measures in case of outbreaks;

iii) advocacy to ensure greater interaction and coordination among national animal and public health systems, and greater engagement between the public and private sectors.

It is critically important to understand that communication cannot replace the provision of services, or overcome structural barriers such as the lack of economic means. Instead, it can use advocacy to influence the provision, availability and uptake of the necessary services, and to encourage the use of subsidies and economic aids available to DAs keepers and producers for promoting and improving bio-security.

Complementary tools for disease prevention and control

Infectious disease prevention and control have three major goals, each of which has one or more methods and tools for achieving it:

1. Find infection fast: surveillance.
2. Kill infected animals quickly and humanely: targeted culling and disposal.
3. Stop infection from spreading: bio-security, vaccination.

Disease prevention and control are most effective and efficient when all three goals are achieved together. Vaccination (under certain circumstances and in conjunction with bio-security), traceability and compartmentalization are all important tools for achieving these goals.

Vaccination programmes

Vaccines are available for many major infectious diseases, including FMD and CSF, but not ASF. Vaccination reduces the pressure of pathogens, shedding and disease pressure in the region. The use of vaccines must be controlled. Recommended vaccines must have been tested for efficiency, be appropriate to the context and be produced in accordance with existing standards (OIE).

Compartmentalization

Zoning and compartmentalization are disease management strategies that pursue essentially the same objective: to establish animal populations with distinct health status, based on effective separation of populations of different status and application of bio-security measures to prevent the introduction of infections. Zoning relies more heavily on geographic factors, such as natural or human-made barriers, while compartmentalization focuses more on management and bio-security within the establishments comprising the compartment, to ensure the maintenance of health status.

Pigs are susceptible to a wide range of diseases that affect productivity and the producer's income - whether he/she is a large-scale commercial producer or has only one scavenging pig. The 2009 influenza pandemic, caused by a new strain of swine-origin H1N1, was a timely reminder of the risks for human health related to livestock production - the same DA species, including pigs, that supports the livelihoods and food security of almost a billion people, most of whom are poor. Among the solutions required to minimize the risk of disease spread, the strengthening of bio-security is a priority. It does not reduce the need for appropriate preparedness plans and adequate resources to control disease outbreaks once they occur, but it is proactive, has a preventive impact and enables producers to protect their assets. A thorough knowledge of pig disease epidemiology and the routes of disease transmission has enabled authorities and producers to develop adequate biosecurity measures for the pig production. Some of these measures are applicable across all production systems, while others are not. Each production system requires specific bio-security measures, and although decision-makers should not compromise on public health, the measures to strengthen bio-security in pig production must take into consideration the technical and financial capacity of stakeholders to implement them. The key to changing behaviors /practices in relation to enhanced bio-security lies in people's perceptions of risk and the resources available at the production level. For meaningful change to take place in rural communities, a holistic, multi-sectoral approach is required to identify critical risk points for disease spread and to understand the evolution of diseases in specific environments, the impact of disease on people, and the impact that people have or can have on disease. The promotion of appropriate sustainable bio-security measures goes hand-in-hand with the use of participatory methodologies and a well-designed communication strategy. Further efforts are required to find the appropriate balance between what the private sector can and will voluntarily implement - based on cost:benefit ratios - and the requirements of regulations. Mutual trust between the public and private sectors is essential. In the case of zoonotic diseases, pre-emptive discussions among public health agencies, veterinary services and the pig keepers and pork industry should take place to ensure a holistic understanding and cooperation in the interest of society in general and pig keepers in particular. Strengthened collaboration between public services and the private sector is crucial for better disease control and eradication.

❑❑❑

CHAPTER-10

Summary and Recommendations

The utilization of domestic animals (DAs) products and services is rapidly increasing because of a fast increase in human population and a large proportion of it being now moving to urban areas because of better facilities of education, employment and incomes. Further families becoming nuclear is leading to an increasing demand for foods of higher quality, both nutritionally and in taste and thus having a higher satiety factor. In western countries there is a gradual decline in consumption of red meat (beef and mutton) and there is a greater preference for chicken, pork and rabbit meat. This trend may also arise in India and pig may attain a greater importance in livestock production, particularly for meat in future under intensive management.

Pig is a very efficient in conversion of relatively low quality feed ingredients into high quality protein food which is acceptable to most meat consumers. Although in India, Muslims; the second dominant religious community and also majority of other communities which are otherwise vegetarian, have little consumption of pork. Pork is still a dominant meat among the economically and socially deprived communities who raise a few piglets under free range scavenging conditions and sell them for income or slaughter them on festive occasions for their own consumption of meat. In spite of some efforts by the Central and State Governments in introducing exotic breeds of pigs to be raised as purebreds on the institutional farms for production of purebred or crossbred boars for grading up of indigenous pigs, the total production of pig meat has not shown any serious increase rather there is a decline in population of pigs and thus in poor production.

DA sector in India, as mentioned earlier, is playing an increasingly important role in providing food and nutrition, energy, industrial raw materials and sustainable self-employment and incomes, especially for economically and socially deprived rural people, like small and marginal farmers and landless laborers. Foods of DAs origin are nutritionally better balanced and contain high quality protein with essential amino acids and also possess micro-nutrients, viz. essential vitamins and minerals. Further, animal foods are more balanced, have higher taste and satiety factor.

Exotic breeds of pigs and their crosses are efficient meat producer and can have two to three liters per year, each with ten to twelve piglets and with a good average daily gain, efficiency of feed conversion and carcass yield and quality. Sows are good mothers with a large number of teats and can rear a large litter under proper feeding and management conditions. Utilizing genetically superior breeds, pork production can be highly profitable. Pigs further do not require very costly and environmentally controlled housing facilities like commercial layer/ broiler chicken and can utilize large quantities of agricultural wastes, agro-industrial byproducts and slaughter-house byproducts.

Pig research and development in India is still in a nascent stage relative to other species of livestock. The ICAR had instituted an AICRP on Pigs with a coordinating unit at the Indian Veterinary Research Institute (IVRI), Izatnagar, U.P. The project envisaged raising pigs under intensive feeding and management and involved two exotic breeds and aimed at their improvement through selection and hybridization. The aim was to improve the litter size, litter survival, live weight gains, efficiency of feed conversion and carcass yield and quality. The project was subsequently changed to study indigenous non-descript free range scavenging pigs, both under extensive and intensive management conditions and take up their genetic improvement through selection and hybridization utilizing both indigenous and exotic breeds and thus additive and non-additive genetic variances in and co-variance among important economic characters. The project now aims at improving both the exotic and indigenous breeds of pigs and also undertakes their crossing. The ICAR has established a National Research Center (NRC) on Pigs at Rani, near Guwahati, Assam, which is undertaking fundamental and applied research on different aspects of swine production, developing sustainable management and conservation technologies for indigenous breeds / types and coordinating the multi-locational and multi-disciplinary project on pig production including a mega pig project for production of a large number of piglets for distribution to progressive farmers.

Although no serious efforts for identification, description and evaluation of pig genetic resources in India has been made, a large number of genetic variants / breeds have been identified and described on the basis of their physical conformation, with a little emphasis on production and adaptation characters. These are essentially available in different regions and states of the country and have accordingly been named. As stated earlier, no efforts have been made so far for fuller description and evaluation of these types / breeds for their sustainable management and conservation. Efforts are now being made by the NRC Pig and AICRP units of Pig for identification, description and evaluation of the different breeds in their respective regions and take steps for their sustainable management and conservation.

The indigenous breeds in most regions are generally smaller in size with hairy and black coat color and elongated face with long snout and short ears. They have early sexual maturity, shorter inter-farrowing interval and have reasonably large litter size. Most of the pig types in North-East have been named after the tribe which rears them or the area in which they are reared. Some of the breeds / types are available in more than one location such as Doom is found in Assam and Meghalaya, similarly Naga local are found in Nagaland, Mizo / Zobawka in Mizoram. Physical conformation of some of the breeds has been described by Assam Agricultural University, ICAR Research Complex for NEH region and NRC Pig. Scavenging system and backyard rearing are most common management systems. Scavenging system is more common in Assam where the pigs are let loose for scavenging during the day and are sheltered during night. Backyard rearing system is most common in tribal belt of NE region. The pigs are kept in temporary shelters constructed with locally available material mostly wood logs and bamboos and are protected from rains and snow with a tin roof. The pigs are generally maintained in the backyard for easy handling and feeding on household waste.

Programmes for improving pig production have been undertaken by the Central and State Governments since independence but the major initiatives came in 4th five year plan when the ICAR initiated an AICRP on pigs with the objectives of studying the performance of pure bred exotic breeds. The breeds involved were Landrace and Large White Yorkshire. Centers were located at ANGRAU Tirupati, AAU, Khanapara and JNKVB, Jabalpur and IVRI, Izatnagar. The coordinating unit and a germplasm center was located at IVRI.

Subsequently, Tamilnadu University of Veterinary and Animal Sciences (TANUVAS) and Kerala Agricultural University (KAU), Mannuthy were included. The ICAR Research Complex Goa Center, Birsa Agricultural University (BAU), Ranchi were added in 2000-01 and Central Agricultural University, Izol campus, and Nagaland University were included but JNKVB, Jabalpur unit was discontinued.

During the 4th and 5th five year plan, the project envisaged to study purebred performance of the two exotic breeds viz., Large White Yorkshire at Tirupati and Jabalpur and Landrace at Khanapara and Izatnagar. The project envisaged (i) assessing various genetic parameters of economically important traits related to production, reproduction and efficiency of feed utilization, (ii) to investigate the effect of protein: energy and evolve a low cost/ economic ration and (iii) to study disease incidence and devise suitable control measures.

At the end of 6th plan, it was decided that in the light of larger population of pigs being non-descript and relatively low producing and maintained under scavenging and with little supplementary feed input. These pigs not only have a large population and spread but are of high economic importance to the rural poor. The technical programme was subsequently modified to include crossbreeding with appropriate exotic breeds in addition to studies on performance of indigenous types of pigs under optimum management, undertake crossbreeding of indigenous with exotic breeds and assess the performance in terms of live weight gains, efficiency of feed conversion, carcass yield, carcass quality and reproduction. The project also emphasized on evolving economic pig ration from locally available conventional and non-conventional feed resources. The halfbreds were to be selected for growth rate using economic ration and study incidence of various diseases and effective prophylactic measures.

Subsequently, the programme was changed during the 10th plan and envisaged that in light of small population size and selection being relatively ineffective, male should be replaced to more often to avoid inbreeding. Early weaning at 4 weeks of age should be practiced and piglets raised on nutritionally balanced creep feed. Region based shelter management and integrated farming systems such as crop and pigs and pig and fish should be studied for their economics. Efforts should be made to reduce overall mortality to less than 10% through forecasting disease incidence from meteorological factors and effective steps should be taken for the control of diseases Economic feed formulation based on the local resources should be developed but the feeding of the experimental stock should be on the laid down feed composition.

Subsequently a more detailed work plan for the existing and the new centers proposed to be included, was decided in 2013 and envisaged raising of animals with 75% exotic inheritance, their *inter se* mating and selection. It was envisaged that a minimum 30 breeding sows would be mated with 10 sires (3:1). The sires will arise from each five unrelated sires. The sires will be selected on the basis of an Index combining litter size at birth and weaning, litter weight at birth and weaning and the number of functional teats (a minimum of 6 pairs of functional teats). The selected animals would be further screened cytogenetically for detecting any genetic abnormality and if positive, would not be used for breeding. The selected males should have a live weight of 65 kg at 8 months. The litter size should be at least seven. The performance of the progeny should be studied in each generation to record the effectiveness of selection. AI should be introduced. The project also envisaged studies on nutrition, physiology, management and health to validate the existing feeding regime and evolve suitable location specific production technologies to reduce environmental stress based on temperature humidity index (THI). Infectious diseases should be properly recorded and their consequent mortality and morbidity should be studied.

The project has been able to develop methodology for (i) improving indigenous pigs through selection, (ii) studies on the performance of purebreds and crosses of Landrace and Large Yorkshire with indigenous types with 50% and 75% exotic inheritance and reciprocal crosses of those involving different breeds. It has been observed that exotic breeds of pigs viz Landrace, Large White Yorkshire can be raised successfully and bred under intensive farm management. Genetic improvement in pigs can be brought through selection and /or crossbreeding with exotic breeds. There is an improvement in litter size at birth and weaning and live weight gains up to 32 weeks of age in crossbreds and purebreds. The selection within the indigenous pigs is slow, primarily due to small effective population size used and low intensity of selection, (iii) the crossbreds have bigger litter size, higher growth rate and better efficiency of feed conversion than the indigenous pigs, (iv) there was further improvement in litter size in increase exotic inheritance from 50 % to 75%. (v) pig can be utilized effectively as a component of integrating farming system, and (vi) it was further observed that the crossbreds involving exotic and indigenous breeds have lower back fat thickness and higher percent of lean meat.

Studies on pig management have led to standardization of semen collection and AI technologies using liquid semen, development of automatic feeders, artificial milk feeding to orphaned piglets. Sprinklers for reducing heat stress and avoid wallowing, pressure cleaning system of pig sties and automatic waterers for pigs have been developed.

Nutritional studies have resulted in determining optimum energy and protein content in feed of different breeds and breed crosses and development of economic rations for different production types.

Studies on pig reproduction conducted have showed that the indigenous pigs both descript and non-descript have relatively lower litter size, live weights at different ages, live weight gains and efficiency of feed utilization but have higher lean meat. The crossbred with exotic breeds have improved litter size and survival, have better growth rate and efficiency of feed conversion than the indigenous pigs. The higher grades (75%) exotic inheritance have higher litter size than half breds.

In addition to the research initiatives under AICRP and now additionally at the NRC pigs, there have been initiatives of the different educational, research and development organizations. The initiatives of the TANUVAS on improving the profitability and resource use efficiency has shown that three way synthetic crossbreds involving Large White York Shire male and Land-race females and F1 females bred to Duroc males, resulted in a better performance in terms of body weight gains and carcass yield and quality. The three breed crosses had higher body weight by 4 kg that Large White York Shire at 8 weeks of age, higher efficiency of feed conversion, dressing percentage, lower back fat thickness and higher ham and bacon percentage. Similarly in Kerala, Kerala Livestock Development Board (KLBD) is undertaking the sustainable management of local Angamaly pigs which are highly disease resistance, environmental stress resistance (temperature and humidity). Their crosses with exotic breeds such as Large White and superior indigenous breed have shown substantial improvement in overall performance. The KLDB is maintaining Large White Land Race and Duroc breeds and producing Large White x Land Race crossbred females and breeding them with Duroc to raise three breed crosses for fattening. Some exotic Asiatic breeds like Myanmar crossbred have been introduced to Manipur by indigenous pig breeders.

There are a large number of threats in the sustainable use and conservation in indigenous pig genetic resources, these are related to:

i) Unidentified and non-descript population which would require identification of all known and not known population, their description and evaluation through extensive surveys in their home tracts. The home tract will also have to be characterized in terms of topography, physical environment and vegetation resources. The population has to be characterized and documented and steps taken for the sustainable use and conservation / preservation depending upon the spread and the population size and structure including the current breeding programmes.

ii) The breeding strategy should be evolved to increase effective population size especially the number of sires used and their turn over, use in other population and change every third year, population trends, identify breeds under threat, establish nucleus population either on institutional farms with a representative sample or through an open nucleus involving a large number of herds with the pig keepers and undertaking intensive selection in the nucleus and supplying superior breeding males or their semen for AI. The use of advanced reproduction biotechnologies can help in increasing the population of breeds/ types that are threatened to extinction.

iii) Improving the performance of the available breeds / strains through selection or grading up with superior breed from comparable agro-ecology.

iv) Restricting excessive slaughter to maintain a large breeding population and using a relatively large number of breeding males and their faster turnover both for avoiding inbreeding and making faster genetic improvement.

v) Provision of adequate nutrition, health, management inputs and marketing facilities to sustain the existing production systems and bring further improvement.

There is a need to educate, both the producers and the consumers regarding hygienic pig meat production and ensuring its quality. There is a need for the meat industry being involved in processing realizing the economic, social and nutritional importance of pig meat and undertake intensive research, education and extension activity to develop more effective production and processing technologies for intensive pig production in the country. The current research on description, evaluation, and sustainable management and conservation of different breeds and types of pigs available in the country as well as pooling all the knowledge available nationally and internationally on the pig breeds, and undertaking their genetic improvement and sustainable utilization for economic pig production along with their feeding, management and health interventions, determining appropriate age and weight at slaughter to maximize economic returns and producing quality meat for consumption as unprocessed or processed meat are areas requiring immediate R&D support.

❑❑❑

Further Reading

Amass S F and Baysinger A. 2006. Swine disease transmission and prevention. In B.E. Straw, J.J. Zimmerman, D.J. Taylor and S. D'Allaire (eds.) Diseases of swine, 9th ed. pp. 1075–1098. Oxford, UK, Blackwell.

Anderson E C, Hutchings G H, Mukarati N and Wilkinson PJ. 1998. African swine fever virus infection of the bush pig (*Potamochoerus porcus*) and its significance in the epidemiology of the disease. *Veterinary Microbiology* **62**: 1–15.

Andraud M, Grasland B, Durand B, Cariolet R, Jestin A, Madec F and Rose N. 2008. Quantification of porcine circovirus type 2 (PCV 2) within and between-pen transmission in pigs. *Veterinary Research* **39** **(5)**: 43.

Banik S, Naskar S, Sarma D K and Tamuli M K (eds). 2014. Breeding and management strategies for piggery enterprises for increased productivity and profitability. National Research Centre on Pig (ICAR), Rani, Guwahati-781 131. Pp.237.

Brandt Y, Lang A, Madej A, Rodriguez-Martinez H, Einarsson S. 2006. Impact of ACTH administration on the oviductal sperm reservoir in sows: The local endocrine environment and distribution of spermatozoa. *Animal Reproduction Science* **92**: 107-122.

Brandt Y, Lang A, Madej A, Rodriguez-Martinez H, Einarsson S. 2006. Impact of ACTH during oestrus on the ultrastructure of the spermatozoa and their environment in the tubal reservoir of the postovulatory sow. *Animal Reproduction Science* **93**: 231-245.

Brandt Y, Lundeheim N, Madej A, Rodriguez-Martinez H, Einarsson S. 2007. Effects of ACTH injections during estrus on concentrations and patterns of progesterone, estradiol, LH, and inhibin á and time of ovulation in the sow. *Domestic Animal Endocrinology* **32**: 122-137.

Brandt Y, Madej A, Rodriguez-Martinez H, Einarsson S. 2007. Effects of exogenous ACTH during oestrus on early embryo development and oviductal transport in the sow. *Reproduction in Domestic Animals* **42**: 118-125.

Broom DM. 1991. Animal Welfare: Concepts and measurements. *Journal of Animal Science* **69**: 4167-4175.

Cameron RD, Blackshow AW. 1980. The effect of elevated ambient temperature on spermatogenesis in the boar. *Journal of Reproduction and Fertility* **59(1)**: 173-179.

Cano J P, Dee S A, Deen J, Finnegan C, Murtaugh M P and Pijoan C. 2007. An exploratory study to evaluate the survival of porcine reproductive and respiratory syndrome virus in non-processed pig meat. *Veterinary Record* **160**: 907–908.

Casal J, De Manuel A, Mateu E and Martin M. 2007. Bio-security measures on swine farms in Spain: Perceptions by farmers and their relationship to current on-farm measures. *Preventive Veterinary Medicine* **82**: 138–150.

Cassar G, Kirkwood R N, Seguin M J, Widowski T M, Farzan A, Zanella A J, Friendship R M 2008. Influence of stage of gestation at grouping and presence of boars on farrowing rate and litter size of group-housed sows. *Journal of Swine Health and Production* **16**: 81-85.

Das A, Tamuli M K, Thomas R, Rajkhowa S and Banik S. 2012. Scientific pig production practices. National Research Centre on Pig, Rani, Guwahati. Indian Council of Agricultural Research. pp. 122.

Dee S A, Deen J, Otake S and Pijoan C. 2004. An experimental model to evaluate the role of transport vehicles as a source of transmission of PRRSV to susceptible pigs. *Canadian Journal of Veterinary Research* **68**: 128–133.

Dee S A, Deen J and Pijoan C. 2005. Evaluation of disinfectants for the sanitation of porcine reproductive and respiratory syndrome virus-contaminated transport vehicles at cold temperatures. *Canadian Journal of Veterinary Research* **69**: 64–70.

Dee S A, Deen J and Pijoan C. 2006. An evaluation of an industry-based sanitation protocol for full-size PRRSV-contaminated transport vehicles. *Swine Health Production* **14**: 307–311.

Dee S A, Deen J, Rossow K D Eliason R, Mahlum C, Otake S, Joo H S and Pijoan C. 2003. Mechanical transmission of porcine reproductive and respiratory syndrome virus throughout a coordinated sequence of events during warm weather. *Canadian Journal of Veterinary Research*, **67**: 12–16.

Edwards R L, Omtvedt I T, Turman E J, Stephens D F, Mahoney G W A. 1968. Reproductive performance of gilts following heat stress prior to breeding and in early gestation. *Journal of Reproduction and Fertility* **52**(Suppl): 47-61.

Gloster J H, Hewson D, Mackay T, Garland A, Donaldson A, Mason I and Brown R. 2001. Spread of foot-and-mouth disease from the burning of animal carcasses on open pyres. *Veterinary Record* **148**: 585–586.

Guérin B and Pozzi N. 2005. Viruses in boar semen: detection and clinical as well as epidemiological consequences regarding disease transmission by artificial insemination. *Theriogenology* **63**: 556–572.

Hugh-Jones M. 2006. Biological disasters of animal origin. The role and preparedness of veterinary and public health services. *OIE Science and Technology Reviews*, **25(1)**: 461 pp.

Jensen T B, Baadsgaard N P, Houe H, Toft N and Ostergaard S. 2008. The association between disease and profitability in individual finishing boars at a test station. *Livestock Science* **117**: 101–108.

Karlen G A M, Hemsworth P H, Gonyou H W, Fabrega E, Strom A D, Smits R J. 2007. The welfare of gestating sows in conventional stalls and large groups on deep litter. *Applied Animal Behaviour Science* **105**: 87-101.

Kelley K W. 1988. Cross-talk between the immune and endocrine systems. *Journal of Animal Science* **66**: 2095-2108.

Koketsu Y, Dial G D, Pettigrew J E, Marsh W E, King V L. 1996. Characterization of feed intake patterns during lactation in commercial swine herds. *Journal of Animal Science* **74**: 1202-1210.

Kongsted A G. 2004. Stress and fear as possible mediations of reproduction problems in group housed sows. A review. *Acta Agric Scand Sect A, Anim Sci* **54**: 58-66.

Lemke U, Kaufmann B, Thuy L T, Emrich K Valle Zárate A. 2006. Evaluation of smallholder pig production systems in North Vietnam: Pig production management and pig performances. *Livestock Science* **105**: 229–243.

Madej A, Brandt, Einarsson S. 2009. Endocrine dynamics associated with follicle development in pigs: a review. *Animal Reproduction* **6**: 135-143.

Madej A, Madsen M T, Brandt Y, Kindahl H, Einarsson S. 2005. Stress related effects on reproductive capacity of pigs. *Journal of Animal Feed Science* **14**(Suppl 1): 205-212.

Maes D, Nauwinck H, Rijsselaere T, Mateusen B, Vyt P, de Kruif A and Van Soom A. 2008. Diseases in swine transmitted by AI: an overview. *Theriogenology* **70**: 1337–1345.

Mohan N H, Tamuli M K, Banik S, and Sarma D K. (eds). 2014. Compendium of lead papers and abstracts. National conference on opportunities and strategies for sustainable pig production, December 20 to 21, 2014. Pp.366.

Morrow W E M, O'Quinn P, Barker J, Erickson G, Post K and McCaw M. 1995. Composting as a suitable technique for managing swine mortalities. *Swine health and production* **3**: 236–243.

Munsterhjelm C, Valros A, Heinonen M, Hälli O, Peltoniemi O A T. 2008. Housing during early pregnancy affects fertility and behavior sows. *Reproduction in Domestic Animals* **43**: 584-591.

Nutrient Requirements of Pig. 2013. Indian Council of Agricultural Research, New Delhi.pp. 22.

Olsen C W, Brown I H, Easterday B C and Van Reeth K. 2006. Swine influenza. *In* B.E.Straw, J.J. Zimmerman, D.J. Taylor and S. D'Allaire, eds. *Diseases of swine*, pp. 469–482.Oxford, UK, Blackwell.

Omtvedt I T, Nelson R E, Edwards R L, Stephens D F, Turman E J. 1971. Influence of heat stress during early, mid and late pregnancy of gilts. *Journal of Animal Science* **32**: 312-317.

Pankaj P K, Pourouchottamane R, Das A, Naskar S, Banik S and Tamuli M K (eds). 2012. Good management practices for improved pig production. National Research Centre on Pig, Rani, Guwahati. Indian Council of Agricultural Research, - 781 131. pp.242.

Payne W J A and Wilson R T. 1999. An introduction to animal husbandry in the tropics. Oxford, UK, Blackwell. 815 pp.

Peters, D. 2005. Rural income generation through improving crop-based pig production systems in Vietnam: Diagnostics and dissemination. *Agriculture and Human Values* **22:** 73–85.

Pinto J C and Urcelay S V. 2003. Biosecurity practices on intensive pig production systems in Chile. *Preventive Veterinary Medicine* **59**: 139–145.

Pitkin A N, Deen J and Dee S A. 2009. Use of a production region model to assess the airborne spread of porcine reproductive and respiratory syndrome virus. *Veterinary Microbiology* **136**:1–7.

Pourouchottamane R, Pankaj P K, Das A, Naskar S, Banik S, Tamuli M K. (eds) 2012. Shelter management for pig rearers in north-east India. National research Centre on Pig, Rani, Guwahati, Indian Council of Agricultural Research. pp.105.

Prunier A, Messias de Braganca M, Le Dividich L. 1997. Influence of high ambient temperature on performance of reproductive sows. *Livestock Production Science* **52**: 123-133.

Radostits O M. 2001. Control of infectious diseases of food-producing animals. Herd health: food animal production medicine, 3rd ed. Philadelphia, Pennsylvania, USA, WB Saunders.

Razdan P, Tummaruk P, Kindahl H, Rodriguez-Martinez H, Hultén F, Einarsson S. 2004 Hormonal profiles and embryo survival of sows subjected to induced stress during days 13 and 14 of pregnancy. *Animal Reproduction Science* **81**: 295-312.

Razdan P, Tummaruk P, Kindahl H, Rodriguez-Martinez H, Hultén F, Einarsson S. 2004. The impact of induced stress during days 13 and 14 of pregnancy on the composition of allantoic fluid and conceptus development in sows. *Theriogenology* **61**: 757-767.

Roozen A W M, Tsuma V T, Magnusson U. 1995. Effects of short-term stress on plasma concentrations of catecholamines, â-endorphin, and cortisol in gilts. *American Journal of Veterinary Research* **56(9):** 1225-1227.

Rougoor C W, Dijkhuisen A A, Huirne R B M and Marsh W E. 1996. Impact of different approaches to calculate the economics of disease in pig farming. *Preventive Veterinary Medicine* **26:** 315–328.

Soede N M, Roelofs J B, Verheijen R J E, Schouten W P G, Hazeleger W, Kemp B. 2007. Effect of repeated stress treatments during the follicular phase and early pregnancy on reproductive performance of gilts. *Reproduction in Domestic Animals* **42**: 135-142.

Suriyasomboon A, Lundeheim N, Kunavongkrit A, Einarsson S. 2004. Effect of temperature and humidity on sperm production in Duroc boars under different housing systems in Thailand. *Livestock Production Science* **89**: 19-31.

Suriyasomboon A, Lundeheim N, Kunavongkrit A, Einarsson S. 2005. Effect of temperature and humidity on sperm morphology in Duroc boars under different housing systems in Thailand. *The Journal of Veterinary Medical Science* **67**: 777-785.

Suriyasomboon A, Lundeheim N, Kunavongkrit A, Einarsson S. 2006. Effect of temperature and humidity on reproductive performance of crossbred sows in Thailand. *Theriogenology* **65**: 606-628.

Vos C J D, Saatkamp H W and Huirne R B M. 2005. Cost-effectiveness of measures to prevent classical swine fever introduction into the Netherlands. *Preventive Veterinary Medicine* **70:** 235–256.

Wettemann RP, Bazer FW.1985. Influence of environmental temperature on prolificacy of pigs. *Journal of Reproduction and Fertility (Suppl)* **33**: 199-208.

Wettemann R P, Wells M E, Omstvedt I P, Pope C E, Turman E J. 1976. Influence of elevated ambient temperature on reproductive performance of boars. *Journal of Animal Science* **42**: 664-669.

❑❑❑

About the Authors

Dr. R.M.Acharya
B.V.Sc. & A.H. (Pb), M.S. (Ohio), Ph.D. (Iowa)
Former Deputy Director General (A.S.), ICAR
784, Sector-9, Faridabad, 121 006, Haryana, India

Dr. R. M. Acharya was associated with National Commission on Agriculture as Member Secretary on the groups on Small Ruminant Production, and Veterinary, Animal Science and Dairy Education and prepared the reports and the recommendation for consideration and acceptance of the commission. The long experience in teaching at undergraduate and postgraduate level in the Punjab/ Haryana Agriculture Universities, research and research management experience at the Universities and under the Indian Council of Agricultural Research as Director, Central Sheep and Wool Research Institute from 1970-1980, which saw tremendous growth of infrastructure and initiation of new initiatives such as AICRPs on Goat for Meat. In position as Deputy Director General (Animal Sciences) was responsible for planning, evaluation and co-ordination of projects in Animal Production, Animal Health and Animal Products Technology, Fisheries Sciences, Social Sciences and Economics and Forage Research. He was member of the FAO expert panels on Animal Genetic Resource Conservation, Biotechnology, Small Ruminant Production and prepared technical bulletins on Sheep and Goat Breeds in India and State of Indian Livestock Genetic Resources. He Was also associated with UNDP, SDC, IDRC, World Bank, Ford Foundation and Rockefeller Foundation on preparation/ evaluation of research and development projects in Animal Husbandry.

Dr. Puneet Kumar
Ph.D.; PGD in Technology Management in Agriculture
Principal Scientist, Animal Physiology and Incharge, Zonal Technology Management Centre, Indian Veterinary Research Institute (IVRI), Izatnagar-243 122, Bareilly (UP), India

Dr. Puneet Kumar served as scientist at Central Institute for Research on Goats, Makhdoom, P.O. Farah, Mathura (UP) for 25 years. There he worked on economical and comfortable animal housing for different agro-climatic conditions, micro-climate and its effect on animal production. He also worked extensively on thermoregulatory mechanisms of goats in different thermal, solar radiation environment coupled with water scarcity. Presently he is working in the area of climate change and its impact on livestock production and diseases at the Indian Veterinary Research Institute, Izatnagar. In addition to research work in Animal Physiology, he is actively engaged in a new initiative of Indian Council of Agricultural Research in the area of Technology Commercialization, Entrepreneurship Development, Intellectual Property Management, Contract and Consultancy Projects through Zonal Technology Management Centre.